ABC OF SPORTS MEDICINE

2nd edition

edited by

GREG McLATCHIE

Visiting Professor of Sports Medicine and Surgical Sciences, University of Sunderland
Consultant Surgeon at Hartlepool General Hospital, and
Director of the National Sports Medicine Institute, London

MARK HARRIES

Consultant Physician at Northwick Park Hospital, Harrow, and Director of Clinical Services,
British Olympic Medical Centre, Harrow

CLYDE WILLIAMS

Professor of Sport and Exercise Science,
University of Loughborough

JOHN KING

Director of the Academic Department of Sports Medicine,
London Hospital Medical College
Consultant Orthopaedic Surgeon, Royal London Hospital, and
Chairman of the British Association of Sport and Medicine

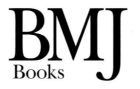

BMJ Books

©BMJ Books 2000
BMJ Books is an imprint of the BMJ Publishing Group

First published in 1995
by BMJ Publishing Group, BMA House, Tavistock Square, London WC1H 9JR
First published 1995
Second impression 1997
Third impression 1998
Second edition 2000
Second impression 2000
Third impression 2001
www.bmjbooks.com

British Library Cataloguing in Publication Data

A catalogue record for this book is available from the British Library

ISBN 0-7279-1366-2

Typeset by Academic Publishing Services,
and printed and bound by Tenon & Polert Colour Scanning Ltd, Hong Kong

Contents

Contributors

I W R Anderson
Consultant in Accident and Emergency, The Victoria Infirmary NHS Trust, Longside Road, Glasgow

David J Ball
Professor of Risk Management, Middlesex University, London

Malcolm W Brown
Director of Medical Services, UK Athletics, 10, Boundary Park, Neston, South Wirral, Cheshire

Richard Budgett
Medical Director, British Olympic Association, and Medical Officer, British Olympic Medical Centre, Northwick Park Hospital, Harrow, Middlesex

Andrea Daly
Boots Teacher/Practitioner in Pharmacy Practice, 407, Water Gardens, Gibralter

Susie Dinan
Senior Clinical Exercise Practitioner, Royal Free Hospital, Pond Street, London

J D M Douglas
Tweeddale Medical Practice, High Street, Fort William, Inverness-shire

Jane Gibson
Consultant Physician, Rheumatic Disease Centre, George Sharp Unit, Cameron Hospital, Windygate, Fife

O J A Gilmore
Consultant Surgeon, The Groin Clinic, Harley Street, London

Richard Godfrey
Chief Physiologist, British Olympic Medical Centre, Northwick Park Hospital, Watford Road, Harrow, Middlesex

J F Goodwin
Emeritus Professor of Cardiology, Royal Postgraduate Medical School, Hammersmith, London

Mark Harries
Consultant Physician, British Olympic Medical Centre, Northwick Park Hospital, Watford Road, Harrow, Middlesex

W Stewart Hillis
Professor of Cardiovascular and Exercise Medicine, Division of Cardiovascular and Exercise Medicine, University of Glasgow, Department of Medicine and Therapeutics, Gardiner Institute, Western Infirmary, Glasgow

Bryan Jennett
Emeritus Professor of Neurosurgery, University of Glasgow. Correspondence to Professor G R McLatchie, North Tees and Hartlepool NHS Trust

Pekka Kannus
Specialist in Sports Medicine, Tampere Research Center of Sports Medicine, The Urho Kaleva Kekkonen Institute for Health Promotion Research, Tampere, Finland

J B King
Consultant Orthopaedic Surgeon, The London Independent Hospital, 1 Beaumont Square, Stepney Green, London

Vijay Kurup
Specialist Registrar in General Surgery, Department of Surgery, North Tees and Hartlepool NHS Trust

Caroline J MacEwen
Consultant Ophthalmologist, Ninewells Hospital and Medical School, Dundee

J MacLean
Research Fellow, Department of Medicine and Therapeutics, University of Glasgow at the Gardiner Institute, Western Infirmary, Glasgow

M F Macnicol
Consultant Orthopaedic Surgeon, The Murrayfield Hospital, 122 Corstorphine Road, Edinburgh

P D McIntyre
Career Registrar, Department of Medicine and Therapeutics, University of Glasgow at the Gardiner Institute, Western Infirmary, Glasgow

W J McKenna
Professor of Cardiology, Department of Cardiological Sciences, St Georges Hospital Medical School, London

Greg McLatchie
Professor of Sports Medicine, University of Sunderland, Consultant Surgeon, North Tees and Hartlepool NHS Trust

N Matthews
Physiotherapist, West Hartlepool Rugby Football Club, Brierton Lane, Hartlepool

R J Maughan
University Medical School, University of Aberdeen, Department of Biomedical Sciences, Foresterhill, Aberdeen

Geoffrey Pasvol
Professor of Infection and Tropical Medicine, Imperial College School of Medicine, Department of Infection and Tropical Medicine, Northwick Park Hospital, Harrow, Middlesex

K R Postlethwaite
Department of Oral and Maxillofacial Surgery, Newcastle General Hospital, Acute Services, Westgate Road, Newcastle upon Tyne

ABC of Sports Medicine

Thomas Reilly
Research Institute for Sport and Exercise Sciences, Liverpool John Moores University, Trueman Building, Webster Street, Liverpool

Patrick S Sharp
Consultant Physician, Department of Diabetes and Endocrinology, Northwick Park and St Mark's NHS Trust, Watford Road, Harrow, Middlesex

A D J Webborn
Sports Physician, Esperance Private Hospital, Hartington Place, Eastbourne, East Sussex

Clyde Williams
Professor of Sports Science, Loughborough University, Department of Physical Education, Sports Science and Recreation Management, Loughborough, Leicestershire

Archie Young
Professor of Geriatric Medicine, University of Edinburgh, 21 Chalmers Street, Edinburgh

1　Nature, prevention and management of injury

Pekka Kannus

Nature of sports injury

Currently, a certain amount of physical activity is considered an important element in health promotion and public interest in health enhancing physical activities, including sports, is increasing. Interest in sporting activities has also grown because of a general increase in leisure time and the availability of various forms of recreational and competitive sports. In competitive sports, training and competition have intensified with a trend towards professionalism.

The consequent upsurge in sporting activity and the intensity of training has caused a corresponding increase in sports injuries, both from acute and overuse trauma. The present number of acute sports injuries treated in hospitals is well documented. Forty years ago, sports injuries comprised 1–2% of all injuries seen in an emergency room, while in the 1970s this figure varied between 5 and 7%. At present about 10% of all hospital-admitted injuries are sustained in sports. These numbers do not represent the real incidence of acute sports injuries, but rather the most severe cases.

With regard to overuse injuries, exact incidence rates are even more difficult to uncover. Definition is uncertain, diagnosis is more difficult to establish, and the population at risk is nearly always unknown. In addition, these injuries are treated independently in different places by different professional and semi-professional persons. The only certain element is that, due to the general increase in sporting activities, the number of overuse injuries has increased dramatically during recent decades. Claims about the relative increase (increase in the incidence) have remained without scientific evidence.

Acute and overuse sports injuries are generally considered to be of a relatively mild character; contusions, strains, and sprains making up as much as 90% of sports related injuries. It is estimated that up to 75% of all sports injuries can be classified as mild to moderate, requiring little, if any, sick leave and absence from sports. The number of injured requiring further treatment as in-patients because of sports injury appears to be around 10%. Furthermore, the number of patients needing operative treatment for acute or overuse injury varies from 5 to 10%.

Although many sports injuries are mild or moderate, treatment of injured athletes often requires special judgement and experience. The attending doctor should have not only special knowledge in sports medicine, but also be familiar with the sport and its rules and demands. A correct diagnosis, immediate treatment, and an effective rehabilitation programme are prerequisites for come-back to the sports arena. Generally, only 100% recovery from injury ensures successful return to sports, while in ordinary patient care the requirements are usually not so strict, for example, in terms of return to work.

Despite advanced knowledge, modern technology, and improved skills in sports medicine, many patients fail to return.

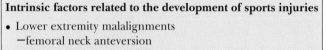

Intrinsic factors related to the development of sports injuries

- Lower extremity malalignments
  - femoral neck anteversion
  - high or low riding patella
  - genu valgum or varum
  - tibia vara
  - pes planus or cavus
  - hindfoot varus or valgus
  - forefoot varus or valgus
  - ankle hyperpronation or hypopronation
- Leg length discrepancy
- Muscle weakness or imbalance
- Decreased flexibility
- Joint hyperlaxity
- Female gender
- Young or old age
- Overweight (obesity)
- Predisposing diseases

Intrinsic factors refer to the makeup of an individual person

Therefore, the prevention of injuries should be a major goal for every doctor and other staff working in the field of sports medicine.

Prevention of sports injury

Sports injuries result from a complex interaction of identifiable risk factors at a given point in time. Since many factors, extrinsic or intrinsic by nature, are involved, the prevention of sports injuries is a complex problem, and a continuing challenge to preventive medicine. In acute sports injuries, extrinsic factors play a major role, while in overuse injuries the reasons are more multifactorial, and interaction between these two categories is common. However, in order to achieve effective injury prevention, it is vital to be able to affect these predisposing risk factors.

Types of injury prevention
In general terms, sports injury prevention refers to all efforts to prevent injuries occurring in connection with sports and physical activity. These efforts can be done at individual, group, or society level (*Figure 1.1*).

Primary prevention
The direct or indirect sports injury prevention at individual level can be called "primary prevention", as is often the case in the prevention strategies in general medicine and health education. Typical examples of primary prevention in sports medicine are: medical preseason or precompetition examination of a subject; warming up before the competition; cooling down after the performance; preventive muscle conditioning; mobility and flexibility training (*Figure 1.2*); coordination and proprioceptive training; sports-specific training; correction of alignment abnormalities in the lower limbs by foot orthotics; proper nutrition, diet, and body hygiene; avoiding too fast a progression in training frequency and intensity, and abrupt changes in training methods; avoidance of doping, unnecessary drugs, and overweight; use of protective equipment, such as helmets, face guards, gum shields, harness, paddings, safety-release ski bindings, braces, or tape (*Figures 1.2* and *1.3*).

In general medicine, an example of primary prevention of lung cancer is an individual decision to stop smoking, or in prevention of atherosclerosis, a decision to reduce the consumption of fatty foods rich in cholesterol.

Secondary prevention
Sports injury prevention at group level can be called "secondary prevention". The most usual way to carry out secondary prevention is group information and education. Lectures to athletes and coaches about the importance of proper warm-up and cooling down, careful following of the rules (fair play), disadvantages of drugs, alcohol and tobacco, and known risk factors of injuries are typical examples. Any decision within individual sport events, which make that particular sport safer, can also be seen as secondary prevention. For example, in prevention of cold injuries in downhill skiing, the demand to cancel a competition because the weather is too cold or windy is a secondary prevention effort.

Respecting lung cancer and atherosclerosis, a public information campaign against smoking, fatty foods, and unhealthy eating habits using television, radio, newspapers, magazines and other mass media is a good way to accomplish secondary prevention.

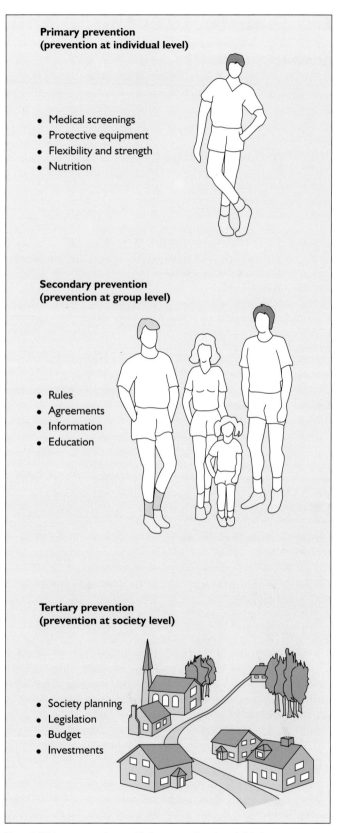

Figure 1.1 Primary, secondary, and tertiary prevention of sports injuries

Tertiary prevention

All efforts undertaken at a society level to prevent sports injuries can be called "tertiary prevention". Normally, tertiary prevention looks a long time ahead and its consequences will not be seen until many years after strategies were planned and put into effect. Society planning is often seen as a tool in tertiary prevention. Concerning sports injury prevention, an example might be a political decision to build new, safe biking routes to the area and keep these completely separate from motor vehicle traffic. Passing legislation to ban all hits to the head in boxing, or full-contact hits or kicks in karate and related combat sports, can be seen as a tertiary effort of prevention.

In prevention of lung cancer, a typical tertiary action is the decision to increase the price of a packet of cigarettes. In atherosclerosis, a government decision to lower the prices of low-cholesterol products, such as fruits and vegetables, and to improve their public availability throughout the year can be viewed as a tertiary preventive measure.

Management of sports injury

Frequently, a sports-related injury is an acute trauma or overuse-induced pain state in the musculoskeletal system of a human body. Since these two injury categories show obvious differences, their management also differs. However, in both acute and overuse injuries, successful management usually requires that a correct and definite diagnosis has been made through a careful history and detailed clinical examination and, if necessary, using radiological techniques, such as radiographs, ultrasound, bone scans, computed tomography, and magnetic resonance imaging.

Management of acute sports injuries

The management of acute musculoskeletal sporting injuries can be divided into two phases: (1) the initial management, or first aid, given immediately after the injury, and (2) further treatment that may consist of surgery and postoperative rehabilitation. Alternatively, the further and more frequent treatment is non-operative, using early controlled mobilisation and functional rehabilitation of the injured body part instead of cast immobilisation.

Initial management

Basic first aid of an acute musculoskeletal sports injury can be remembered by the acronym PRICES: protection, rest, ice, compression, elevation, and support (*Figure 1.4*). Protection refers to all precautions that protect the athlete from making the injury worse, including stopping the causative activity and supporting the injured area. Rest is necessary in the acute phase of the injury to avoid prolonging the acute inflammatory phase; complete rest should be prescribed initially, followed by partial rest later in the rehabilitation process. Rest usually refers to the part of the body that is injured, not the entire athlete. Ice is used to control pain, inflammation, bleeding, and oedema, and to prevent further damage at the site of the injury. Compression is needed for support and for decreasing oedema. Elevation also helps to decrease the oedema by decreasing blood flow in the injured area. Support by cast, brace, splint, or wrap helps to stabilise the injured part of the body and to prevent further damage.

Figure 1.2 Regular stretching and flexibility training and use of protective equipment by a junior ice hockey goalkeeper are excellent examples of primary or individual level prevention of sports injuries

---

Extrinsic factors related to the development of sports injuries

- Training errors
  - high intensity or volume
  - over distance
  - fast progression
  - hill work
  - fatigue
  - non-optimal technique
- Excessive load on the body
  - number of repetitions
  - type and speed of movement
  - surface
  - footwear
- Environmental malconditions
  - wind
  - dark
  - heat or cold
  - humidity
  - altitude
- Poor equipment
  - worn shoes, faulty rackets
  - non-adjusted ski boot bindings
- Ineffective rules
  - violent play

Extrinsic factors refer to all factors that affect externally on the human body

---

The basic first aid of an acute musculoskeletal injury according to the acronym PRICES

P = Protection of the injured area from further damage

R = Rest of the injured part to avoid prolonging irritation

I = Ice for controlling pain, bleeding and oedema

C = Compression for support and controlling swelling

E = Elevation for decreasing bleeding and oedema

S = Support for stabilisation of the injured part

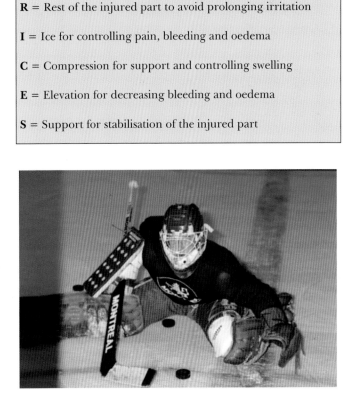

This initial management of an acute sports injury is continued through the entire inflammatory phase of healing (the first 4–7 days) or, if early surgery is planned, until the injured athlete is in the operating theatre.

Further treatment

Although complete muscle, tendon, and ligament ruptures often require early surgical correction in younger competitive athletes, a non-operative treatment with well supervised rehabilitation may be an acceptable primary alternative in older recreational athletes. In the latter group, persistent functional deficit and the level of aggravation experienced by the individual determine if delayed repairs or late reconstruction are needed. In milder strains, sprains, and partial tears of the above noted tissues, nonoperative treatment is the rule, and surgery is performed in the most chronic pain states and conditions only.

During the proliferative phase (7–21 days) and the maturation and remodelling phase of tissue healing (3–8 weeks, and sometimes up to 12 months), the non-operative further treatment of an acute sports injury may use movement and exercise (rehabilitation), anti-inflammatory medication, heat, ultrasound and electrical stimulation to promote healing. If the condition becomes chronic, the non-operative treatment may also include some forms of treatment for chronic overuse injuries, such as corticosteroid-anesthetic injections and massage.

Management of overuse injuries

Acute (inflammatory) conditions

An acute inflammatory response is the body's reaction to a single or repeated insult, or an injury or other destructive factor. Inflammation is manifested in insulted tissues as swelling, erythema, increased temperature, pain, and loss of function.

Initial control of inflammation is best achieved by decreasing activity and by rest, mild compression, cold and anti-inflammatory medication. Decreasing the intensity, frequency and duration of the activity that caused the overuse injury, or modification of that activity, may be the only necessary measure to control the inflammation in the acute phase. Mild compression provided by wrapping may also help to control swelling and pain.

A more specific treatment modality of acute inflammation includes ice or other types of cryotherapy (such as cold compresses, ice or snow packs, ice massage, ice immersion, and gel refrigerant packs) and remains the single, most useful, intervention. Cold can control pain and oedema as well as reduce regional blood flow and the metabolic demands of the tissue, thereby helping to prevent further tissue damage at the site of the injury. Cold also has beneficial effects during rehabilitation by decreasing pain and muscle spasm to allow better mobilisation. In clinical practice, cooling of the tissue area with acute inflammation should be used intermittently over the first days (for example, 20–25 minutes at one hour intervals). Cold injuries should be avoided, however, by not using excessive compression and protecting the underlying skin from direct cold pack contact.

The benefit of nonsteroidal anti-inflammatory drugs (NSAIDs) in the form of pills or topical gels is not as obvious as the use of cold. The healing of an acute soft tissue inflammation may be slighly more rapid and the inflammation slightly better controlled with the use of NSAIDs than without them; however, most patients will recover from the acute condition whether or not NSAIDs are given. NSAIDs do have an analgesic effect and are used by many doctors primarily for this indication alone. They also help patients with more chronic overuse injury symptoms to comply with rehabilitation.

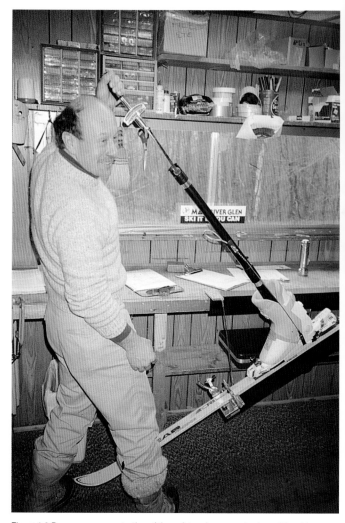

Figure 1.3 Proper preseason testing of the safety-release mechanism of the ski bindings is one way to reduce acute knee ligament injuries in downhill skiing

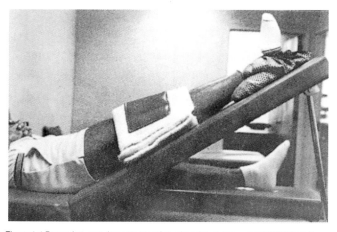

Figure 1.4 Protection, rest, ice, compression, elevation, and support (PRICES) is the correct first aid for an acute knee sprain

The use of corticosteroid-anaesthetic injection therapy in acute subacute inflammation remains controversial. Almost all studies agree that this therapy dramatically affects and alleviates symptoms in synovial and connective tissue structures with prominent immunological and inflammatory activity. They also may inhibit the formation of scar tissue. However, steroid injections, especially if repeated, can be problematic because they may have a deleterious effect on the structure and tensile strength of soft tissues (such as muscle, tendon, and ligament) and thus predispose to rupture.

Finally, correction of the predisposing intrinsic or extrinsic aetiological factors behind the acute inflammation may be critical in preventing the condition from becoming chronic. For example, patients suffering from both tenosynovitis of the posterior tibial tendon, the medial tibial stress syndrome or Achilles peritendinitis, as well as flat-foot deformity and ankle hyperpronation, are likely to benefit from custom-made orthotics that support the medial long arch of the foot, thereby preventing excessive foot pronation (*Figures 1.5a and 1.5b*).

Chronic overuse injuries

Compared with the good consensus on the treatment of acute forms of soft tissue inflammations, there are a variety of suggested therapy modalities for more chronic conditions and the modalities used are frequently only empirically adapted from clinical work without proper scientific support. This is especially true of the use of various modalities of physical therapy and rehabilitation.

The treatment principles of activity modification, rest, cold, NSAIDs, and steroid injections are as described above. Rehabilitation, in terms of stretching and strengthening, is currently seen as one of the most important components in treatment of chronic overuse injuries. The belief in stretching and strengthening as a curative method is based on the concept that, only if the patient can improve the strength and elasticity of the involved tissues to again withstand all the stresses applied on them, will the tissue be able to heal and endure further loads of activity without recurring symptoms. In clinical practice, the initial strengthening exercises are usually isometric followed by the concentric or eccentric dynamic exercises (*Figure 1.6*). The so-called functional rehabilitation, or closed or entire kinetic chain exercises, aimed at rehabilitating the whole limb–body system in a sport-specific way instead of just moving the injured part, have become increasingly popular in the 1990s. In functional rehabilitation, strength, power, endurance, proprioception, balance, and coordination are equally emphasised. Rehabilitation is often guided and supervised by a physiotherapist.

The management of chronic overuse injuries is often reinforced with heat, ultrasound, electrical stimulation, massage, manipulation, mobilisation, and strapping, alone or in combination (*Figure 1.7*). Scientific evidence of their effectiveness is, however, sparse and, especially with regard to clinical evidence, somewhat controversial.

The surgical managent of a chronic overuse injury, such as chronic peritendinitis, insertional tendinitis, tendinosis (tendon degeneration), tenosynovitis, partial tendon tear, or bursitis, has become an acceptable choice in patients who do not adequately respond to conservative treatments (*Figures 1.8a and 1.8b*). In general, surgery has shown good clinical results, although the healing of operated tissue has been seldom verified biochemically, microscopically, functionally, and radiologically. Systematic postoperative rehabilitation is usually regarded as a prerequisite for long-lasting results and prevention of recurrence.

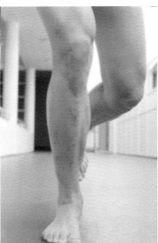
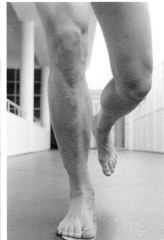

Figure 1.5(a) Hyperpronation of the ankle, external rotation of the tibia and genu valgum are evident in the squatting test of a sportsman

Figure 1.5(b) A custom-made orthotic giving support to the medial arch of the foot prevents all the noted malalignments

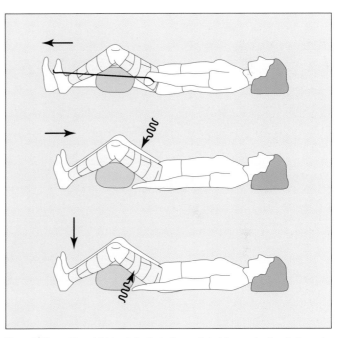

Figure 1.6 Isometric and light resistive isotonic muscle training can be done in the early phase of rehabilitation of various sports injuries

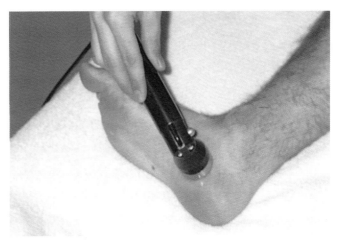

Figure 1.7 Ultrasound management of chronic plantar fasciitis of a middle-aged long distance runner

Summary of the key points

With the increase in sporting activity and intensity there has been an increase in sports injuries, both from acute traumas and overuse symptoms. Sports injuries result from a complex interaction of extrinsic and intrinsic risk factors. The extrinsic factors play a dominant role in acute injuries, while in overuse injuries the reasons are more multifactorial and interaction between these two categories is common.

The management of sports injuries often requires special judgement and experience. The attending doctor needs to have a specialised knowledge in sports medicine and should also be familiar with the sport, its rules and demands. Clarification of the cause(s) of the injury, correct diagnosis, immediate treatment, and effective rehabilitation are often prerequisites for the athlete's come-back to the sports arena. Usually, only 100% recovery from injury ensures a successful return to sports.

Despite advanced knowledge, modern technology, and improved skills in sports medicine, many athletic patients fail to return. Therefore, the prevention of injuries should be a major goal for every doctor and all other staff working in the field of sports medicine.

References

Brukner P, Khan K (1993) *Clinical Sports Medicine*. Blackwell Scientific, Oxford

DeLee JC, Drez Jr. D (1994) *Orthopaedic Sports Medicine*, Vol I and II. WB Saunders, Philadelphia, PA

Józsa L, Kannus P (1997) *Human Tendons. Anatomy, Physiology and Pathology*. Human Kinetics, Champaign, IL

Peterson L, Renström P (1986) *Sports Injuries. Their Prevention and Treatment*. Martin Dunitz, London

Figure 1.8 Surgical treatment of the chronic Achilles insertitis and retrocalcaneal bursitis

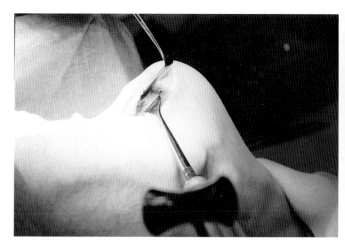

a) After excision of the chronically inflamed bursa, the prominent posterosuperior tuberosity of the calcaneus (Haglund's deformity) is partially resected

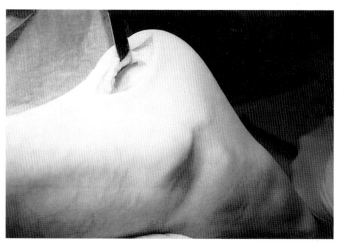

b) The view after the bone resection and before the skin closure

2   Head injury
Vijay Kurup, Greg McLatchie, Bryan Jennett

Most sports related injuries are musculoskeletal, affecting limbs or trunk, and related to specific risks associated with particular sports. Head injuries, by contrast, can occur in many sports and, except those incurred during boxing, are accidental. Unlike other injuries, the effects of which are usually maximal at onset, injury to the head may precipitate a process of intracranial disorder that can convert a mild initial injury into a life-threatening condition from secondary complications. Moreover, even mild injuries are often associated with considerable temporary disability and repeated mild injuries can result in cumulative brain damage. Doctors on sports fields have to decide whether patients with head injuries can resume play or, if not, what further immediate management is needed and when they can play again. The answers to these questions depend on a sensible balancing of risks.

The nature of brain damage

Pathophysiology
Most sports related head injuries are due to blunt trauma. Penetrating injuries are less common. In most cases marked acceleration or deceleration forces are imparted to the head.

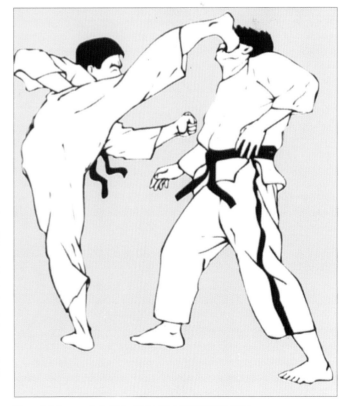

Figure 2.1 In boxing, injuries to the head account for 40% of all injuries. A boxer who sustains three knockouts is not permitted to fight for the rest of the season

Incidence of sporting head injuries in Glasgow requiring neurosurgical admission	
Golf	28%
Horse riding	16%
Football	14%
Shooting	10%
Climbing	8%
Rugby	6%
Boxing	4%

Damage to the brain is the main concern when the head suffers a blow. Injuries to the scalp or skull are only important as indicators of the possibility of underlying impact damage, or of the risk of complications that could cause secondary brain damage.

An open (compound) depressed fracture of the skull vault poses the risk of intracranial infection if formal surgical debridement is not carried out, but the injury may only be regarded as a simple scalp laceration. Infection is also a risk with basal skull fractures penetrating the dura over the nasal sinuses or the middle ear.

Clues to basal fracture are CSF rhinorrhoea or otorrhoea, periorbital ecchymoses (racoon eyes) or retroauricular bruising (Battle's sign).

Figure 2.2 An uncontrolled (illegal) roundhouse kick to the head

Primary brain damage

Impact (or primary) damage can take two forms:

Cerebral contusions

Bruising on the brain surface due to the brain's impact with the overlying skull are the most common form of impact damage. Contusion may be focal underneath a fracture resulting from a focal impact, blunt or penetrating, or it may be diffuse, resulting from the brain as a whole being thrown against the rough interior surface of the skull and dural dividers. Diffuse contusion results when the head as a whole decelerates, usually by hitting the ground, in which case the contusions are usually bilateral, affecting the surfaces of both frontal and temporal lobes regardless of where the head was actually struck. Contusions themselves do not necessarily cause impaired consciousness or focal neurological signs, unless they are over the motor strip, the speech area, or the visual cortex. Their main importance is that they may initiate secondary local brain swelling and continued bleeding may produce an intradural haematoma.

Diffuse axonal injury

This is widespread tearing of the white matter fibres in the subcortical areas of the brain. This can occur without pronounced contusions, or a fracture of the skull and it usually causes immediate unconsciousness, but this can be variable in duration.

Secondary brain damage

This results from three main mechanisms:

Raised intracranial pressure

This results from either an acute intracranial haematoma or brain swelling, often both. A haematoma causes midline shift of the brain with a tentorial herniation causing distortion of the brain stem where secondary haemorrhage eventually has a fatal outcome. Brain swelling is a consequence of vascular engorgement, a cerebral oedema, or both and it may be focal or diffuse. Respiratory obstruction or inadequacy (causing a raised $PaCO_2$ and lowered PaO_2) will cause vasodilatation in the cerebral vessels and subsequent engorgement of the whole brain. It also aggravates any focal swelling around contusions. Oedema of the hemisphere often occurs after surgical removal of an acute intracranial haematoma, especially if this has been delayed.

Hypoxia and ischaemia

Both are found in a high proportion of fatal cases of brain damage and contribute considerably to disability in survivors of severe injuries. The main cause is raised intracranial pressure, which reduces the flow of blood into the skull, but an aggravating factor is lowered blood pressure and haemoglobin content in the blood because of associated extracranial injuries. These are likely to occur in sporting injuries only when the whole body has suffered violence, as in accidents associated with climbing, horse riding, racing cars, or motorcycles.

Intracranial infection

Intracranial infection (meningitis or brain abscess) is a possibility when the dura has been penetrated by injury as described above.

Second impact syndrome (SIS)

SIS has been described as occurring when "an athlete who has sustained an initial head injury, most often concussion, sustains a second head injury before symptoms associated with the first have fully cleared". It is postulated that the second impact predisposes to the rapid development of cerebrovascular congestion, which, in turn, raises intracranial pressure resulting in brain stem herniation and death. Boxers, children and adolescent males are predicted to be at high risk. Fortunately, the incidence is very low.

Clinical features and action required:
(see Glasgow coma score)

The Glasgow coma score

Eye opening

Spontaneous	4
To voice	3
To pain	2
None	1

Best verbal response

Orientated	5
Confused	4
Inappropriate words	3
Incomprehensible	2
None	1

Best motor response

Obeys commands	6
Localises pain	5
Withdraws from pain	4
Flexes to pain	3
Extends to pain	2
None	1

Possible total	(range)	3–15

Altered consciousness

Altered consciousness is the hallmark of diffuse brain damage. It is evidenced by immediate change in responsiveness and in subsequent loss of memory for an interval after injury—post-traumatic amnesia (PTA). The Glasgow coma scale is now the accepted means of assessing patients with head injuries for signs of deterioration that would indicate complications calling for immediate action, both initially and for continued observations. Most head injuries are mild, resulting in only a minute or so of eyes-closed coma with no speech and not obeying commands. As a player regains consciousness, the important observation is whether there is a rapid return to full orientation in person, time and place. Those who have been completely knocked out and some who have only been dazed will have a period of incomplete recovery, during which automatic behaviour may enable them to continue playing, but of which period they have no subsequent memory. When there has been a definite period of coma, the post-traumatic amnesia always extends for a considerable time after return to responsive behaviour, and the duration of amnesia is considered the best guide to the severity of diffuse brain damage. Some years ago, a study of 544 rugby footballers in Britain found 56% had suffered at least one head injury associated with post-traumatic amnesia; this had lasted more than an hour in 58 players, of whom only 38 had been admitted to hospital for observation.

Concussion

In America, several competing systems for grading mild head injuries have been developed, mainly as a guide to when sport may be resumed. They are usually called grades of concussion and they have been widely adopted in sports medicine, although not used in other contexts.

Mild concussion (Grade I)

This is an injury where consciousness is preserved, but there will be associated temporary neurological dysfunction. These are the most common injuries and often go unnoticed because of the trivial nature of symptoms. Common symptoms include confusion, disorientation, headache and photophobia. These are nearly always associated with post-traumatic amnesia, but this lasts less than 30 minutes. Usually, these symptoms are completely reversible.

Moderate concussion (Grade II)
There will be associated loss of consciousness (less than 5 minutes) and both retrograde and post-traumatic amnesia (memory loss regarding events immediately before and for some time after the injury), together with symptoms described in Grade I.

Severe concussion (Grade III)
Here the causative injury is much more severe and invariably associated with loss of consciousness and post-traumatic amnesia that lasts longer. The loss of consciousness is reversible and the norm is to return to consciousness within six hours. However, the duration of post-traumatic amnesia can vary and the length of amnesia is proportional to the severity of the injury. Retrograde amnesia is a less reliable tool than post-traumatic amnesia in assessing the severity of the injury.

In some patients who suffer severe concussion recovery is often incomplete and leaves long-standing neurological deficits and other symptoms, such as dizziness, depression, nausea, anosmia, chronic headache, fatigue, and sleep disturbance. These are collectively referred to as the post-concussion syndrome and can be very disabling.

Field assessment of players with head injuries
Scalp wounds often lead to brisk bleeding and players should be removed for careful inspection of the wound and control of

Neurological history
This will be obtained from the doctor's own observations, witnesses, the ambulance crew, or other emergency service staff:
1 What were the circumstances of the accident (tackle, scrum collapse, fall, etc)?
2 Has the patient talked at any time?
3 What was the patient's Glasgow coma score at the accident scene?
4 Has the patient's Glasgow coma score altered en route?
5 Has the patient taken alcohol or any other drugs?
6 Has the patient had a fit?

Neurological examination
• Glasgow coma scale
• Pupil sizes and responses to light
• Examination of ears and nose for blood, cerbrospinal fluid and haemotympanum
• Sensation (including the perianal area)
• Deep tendon reflexes (including plantar responses)
• Movement of all limbs to assess motor function

Grading the severity of cerebral concussion

Symptom	Grade I (mild)	Grade II (moderate)	Grade III (severe)
Post-traumatic amnesia	<30 minutes	>30 minutes and <24 hours	>24 hours
Loss of consciousness	None	<5 minutes	>5 minutes

haemorrhage. Such players are not permitted to stay on the field because of the risk of transmitting HIV. The wound may then be assessed with a sterile gloved finger to assess whether there is a fracture. This is often easier to feel than see. Patients with compound depressed fractures of the vault suffer only local brain damage and, as they often do not lose consciousness, the potential seriousness of the injury can be overlooked. Scalp wounds in sport are most commonly the result of being struck by a golf club or ball, billiards cue, bat, or racket.

If there is evident herniation of brain tissue through the skull the wound should be covered with a dressing soaked in sterile saline and immediate transport for neurological care or advice arranged. Patients with suspected fractures should first have bleeding controlled by closing the scalp with through and through interrupted sutures before transport to hospital. Minor cuts, however, can be sutured and, providing the wound can be covered, the player may return to the field if fully conscious.

The doctor should have witnessed the incident and when called on to the field by the referee should ask the player appropriate questions, for example, "What happened to you?", "What is the score?", "Where are you?" If the doctor knows the player well then questions relating to family, home or possessions may indicate whether confusion is present. Eye opening and

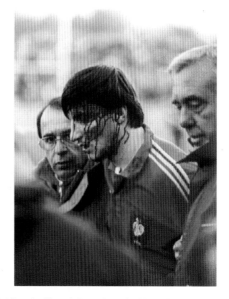

Figure 2.3 People with scalp lacerations should be referred to hospital for radiology for possible skull fracture

pupillary size and response to light can also be observed at this initial assessment.

Some field tests, such as finger to nose, finger to finger, or asking the patient to move certain limbs, may assess the best motor response. Equilibrium is often impaired after concussion. Heel to toe standing with the eyes open or closed is not possible in 35% of such players, and standing on one foot with the other suspended is not possible in 50% (the foot on the ground moves or the suspended foot touches the ground). Unfortunately, false positive results also occur, but these tests may indicate the need for more detailed examination in the medical room.

If the player has not lost consciousness and has full memory of the event, he or she may continue to play. It should, however, be a rule to send off any player who does not immediately regain full consciousness and orientation. Players with post-traumatic amnesia are at risk of further injury if allowed to play on because their automatic behaviour may not allow them to protect themselves as efficiently as they normally would.

A more difficult decision is what further management players or contestants with head injuries need. They should be referred to hospital if they are still confused after ten minutes or so. That would also apply to those in whom an open injury is suspected because of a scalp laceration or blood and fluid coming from the nose or ears. The accident and emergency department can then decide whether a skull X-ray is required to exclude a skull fracture.

If a vault fracture is found, the patient will need to be kept in for observation and probable computed tomography, because the risk of an **acute intracranial haematoma** is considerably increased if there is a vault fracture. Over half the patients with acute intracranial haematomas requiring surgery had been walking and talking when first seen at hospital and some 15% had remained orientated ever since their accident. Delay in recognising and removing an acute intracranial haematoma is the most common cause of avoidable mortality and morbidity after head injury. In sports medicine it is, therefore, important to ensure that any player with a head injury, who goes home from an away or a home game, is continuously accompanied by a colleague who can observe whether there is any change in the level of consciousness (for example, becoming confused), complaints of increasing headache, or vomiting. Family and friends should be informed of the need to maintain this observation. The occurrence of any of these features calls for immediate referral to hospital (even if the player has already been seen and discharged from hospital).

Accident and emergency departments sending home patients with head injuries now usually give the family or accompanying people a head injury card with these instructions. Sports organisations could make use of such a card, which includes the telephone number of the local hospital. Players who have sustained head injuries should avoid alcohol for at least the next 24 hours because they will probably be unduly susceptible to its effects and also because it may lead to confusion in interpreting symptoms that could indicate complications.

After more severe injuries, the possibility of **extracranial injuries** should always be considered, because these are easily overlooked in comatose patients who cannot draw attention to them. Cervical spine fractures, chest and abdominal injuries, and limb fractures all need to be looked for. Suspected cervical spine fractures require splintage initially with manual in-line stabilisation. The patient should be supine and the head in the neutral position. The attendant grasps the mastoid processes and a semi-rigid collar can then be applied (for example, the Philadelphia/Stifneck). Unconscious patients to be transported from the scene of injury require care to avoid airway obstruction; they should be put in the semi-prone coma position until paramedics arrive and can institute suction and intubation. If

Head injury card

- This patient has received an injury to the head. A careful examination has been made and no signs of serious complications has been found
- It is expected that recovery will be rapid, but in such cases it is not possible to be quite certain
- If you notice any change in behaviour, vomiting, dizziness, headache, double vision, excessive drowsiness, please telephone the hospital at once
- No alcohol
- No analgesics
- No driving

Figure 2.4

1) **Mental-Status Testing**

a) Orientation:	Time, place, person and circumstances of injury
b) Concentration:	Digits backwards. Months of year in reverse order.
a) Memory:	Opposite team. Last play called. Recent newsworthy events. Remember 3 words and 3 objects at 0 and 5 minutes.

2) **Neurological Tests**

Pupils:	Symmetry and reaction.
Co-ordination:	Finger–nose test. Finger–nose (eyes closed). Romberg sign.
Sensation:	

3) **Exertional Provocative Tests**

for example, 40 yards sprint
        5 push ups

– any associated symptoms = abnormal result
for example, headache, dizziness, nausea, photophobic blurred vision, emotional lability or mental status change.

Figure 2.5 Sideline evaluation for concussion

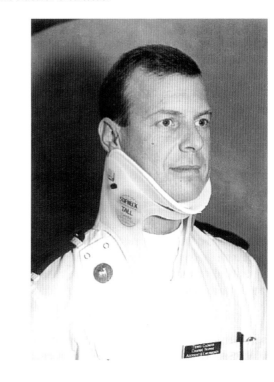

Figure 2.6

intubation is required, an assistant grasps the mastoid processes and the front of the semi-rigid collar can then be safely removed as it can impede mouth opening and does not contribute significantly to neck stabilisation during laryngoscopy.

Manual in-line stabilisation reduces neck movement during intubation, but care must be taken to avoid excessive axial traction that may cause distraction or subluxation. Ideally three or four people are required: the first pre-oxygenates and intubates, the second applies cricoid pressure, the third maintains cervical stabilisation, and the fourth, if present, can give intravenous drugs and assist. Both nasotracheal and orotracheal intubation are given equal emphasis when dealing with patients with suspected cervical spine injury who are unconscious. The use of anaesthetic induction agents and neuromuscular blockers may be given in relation to the experience of the attending physician or paramedic. Nasotracheal intubation in a conscious patient is contraindicated if a basal skull fracture is suspected, or if there is a risk of causing epistaxis vomiting, or regurgitation.

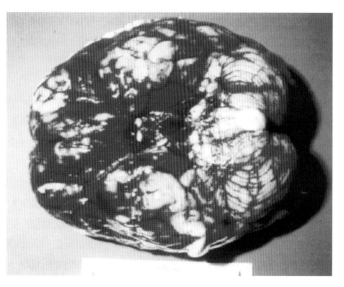

Figure 2.7 Traumatic subarachnoid haemorrhage—the result of an uncontrolled karate roundhouse kick.

Sequelae of head injuries

Injuries that are severe, either initially or because of complications, are often associated with persisting, even permanent effects. Changes in mental function are the most consistent and also the most disabling. These include loss of intellectual capacity, poor recent memory, and personality change. Physical sequelae include hemiparesis, dysphagia, hemianopia, cranial nerve palsies, and traumatic epilepsy.

Mild injuries commonly cause considerable disability for 2–3 weeks. Patients report headaches and dizziness, lack of concentration, fatigue, and difficulties in coping with high level mental functions. These symptoms were once believed to be largely psychological, perhaps motivated by claims for liability, and are rare in athletes. Psychometric tests, however, have now shown clear evidence of impaired information processing for 2–3 weeks after injury. Moreover, athletes often suffer from these symptoms after concussion, although they are less common after severe injury, perhaps because less is expected of them in the early stages of injury. It is, therefore, important to ensure that players with head injury take time off work, but are reassured that these symptoms are expected to be temporary and do not forecast any continuing disability.

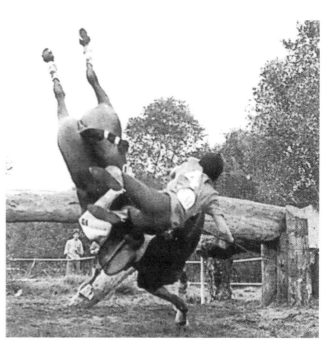

Figure 2.8 In horse riding hats approved to BSI standards must be worn. Multiple injuries can result from falls like this

Return to sport

All participants in contact sports should be required to take three weeks off the sport after a definite head injury and longer if still suffering from symptoms after concussion. There is good evidence that a second injury has a greater effect than an initial one and that repeated injuries, even if mild, can cause cumulative damage. For boxers and horse riders, who are at most risk of repetitive injury, there must come a time when retirement is recommended for those who are often injured. Players of contact sports who have had a craniotomy should probably not play again, as the bone flap can be at risk of displacement.

Details relating to head injury incidents must be recorded in either the club's accident book or the fighter's personal record book. In combat sports, such as boxing, the rest time after a knockout is four weeks. Fighters who are knocked out more than three times a year are suspended for the rest of the season.

Prevention of head injury

Prevention of primary head injury should be the aim, but in sports, such as boxing, this would be extremely difficult to achieve unless there were radical changes in the rules. In non-combative sports, however, most injuries are accidental. In some, such as skateboarding, cycling (leisure cycling in children), horse riding and climbing, head injury can be anticipated and protective headgear should be worn. The age range of youngsters injured while playing golf (from under 16 years in one study) suggests that they should be forewarned of the need to stand well clear when others are wielding golf clubs.

Sports that make use of headgear are increasing in numbers, for example, American football, winter sports, cricket, climbing, cycling, skateboarding, and aerial sports. The value of protective headgear in motorcycle and autosport racing accidents has been well established and in sports such as steeple chase riding, primary serious head injury and cumulative damage have been reduced after these risks were identified. The helmet design used by these jockeys resembles that of a motor cycle helmet. The Pony Club compels competing riders to wear an approved jockey skull cap (BS4472), or a riding hat with a flexible peak (BS6473). Stable lads are not insured unless they wear ND4472 type caps, and a change in attitude towards the use of these by the three million people who ride for pleasure would probably reduce the high incidence of head injuries sustained in riding accidents. Although legislation now requires that young equestrians wear proper protective headgear, fashion is more likely to persuade them to do so. The Young Riders Protective Headgear Act 1990 requires children of 14 years and under to wear an approved hat, suitably harnessed, when riding on a highway.

During boxing training sessions head protection is regularly worn and is now a feature of the Olympic Games. In countries where headgear is compulsory, there has been a reduction in the number of facial cuts and knockouts. Controlling the type of sparring and limiting the number of fights in a boxer's career has been suggested to reduce the risk of cumulative damage. In one survey the risk increased after 40 fights. In addition, the use of padded or sprung flooring protects against serious injury in combat sports.

Prevention of secondary brain damage depends on recognising the risks of certain types of injury and ensuring that medical aid is sought. Some sporting events are attended by a doctor, but in many the referee or trainer must learn what to do. Education in this topic is currently being addressed by the National Coaching Foundation and supported by many of the governing bodies of sport.

References

American College of Surgeons (1997) *ATLS Course Manual 1997*. American College of Surgeons, Chicago, USA

Cantu RC, Micheli LJ (1991) *ACSM's Guidelines for the Team Physician*. Lea and Febiger, Philadelphia

McCrory PR, Beikonia S (1998) *Neurology* **March**: 677–83

Guidelines for return to sports activities after concussion

Grade	First concussion	Second concussion	Third concussion
Grade I (mild)	May return to play if asymptomatic for 1 week	May return to play in 2 weeks if asymptomatic at that time for 1 week	Terminate season; may return to play next season if asymptomatic
Grade II (moderate)	May return to play after asymptomatic for 1 week	After minimum of 1 month, may return to play if asymptomatic for 1 week; consider terminating season	Terminate season; may return to play next season if asymptomatic
Grade III (severe)	After minimum of 1 month, may return to play if asymptomatic for 1 week	Terminate season; may return to play next season if asymptomatic	

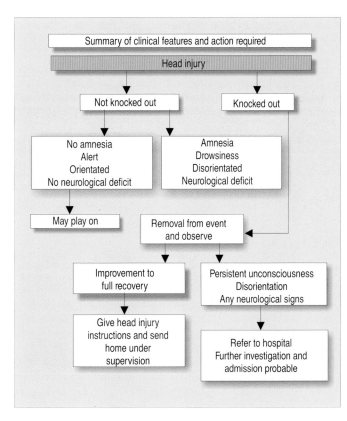

3 Management of the acutely injured joint

J B King

The concept of "management" involves making a diagnosis; far too frequently treatment of injuries to major joints starts without a diagnosis being made.

Whatever diagnostic methods follow in the text, a knowledge of likely injury patterns is a huge help. This, to some extent, is experience, but any opportunity to read or otherwise learn about common injury patterns will make eventual diagnosis so much easier. A good example is the skiing injury in someone approaching a small bump, who is not very experienced. He/she may brace him/herself and feel something pop in the knee, followed by quite rapid swelling. This is the rare but recognised isolated tear of the anterior cruciate ligament brought about by an excessive pull from the quadriceps. This is a specific although not very common example, but the majority of frequently seen injuries do have a pattern; the meniscus tear in full flexion, twisting under load; the shoulder dislocation in forced abduction/external roatation. Get to know the patterns of injury and this will eliminate silly diagnoses, such as a torn anterior cruciate caused by a blow on the front of the flexed knee.

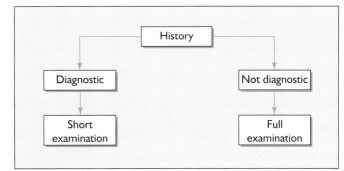

Figure 3.1

Diagnosis

History
In an acute joint injury, it may not always be possible to take a good history, for example, where a scrum has collapsed. However, in many cases the story points to the eventual diagnosis. The fall on the point of the shoulder damages the acromio-clavicular or sternoclavicular joint; the rugby tackle with the leading arm being knocked into external rotation while 90° abducted, points to a shoulder dislocation; the non-contact, twisting, deceleration injury of the knee, followed by a snapping or popping sensation and rapid swelling, is usually associated with a torn anterior cruciate. So history really is important and it is well worth the time spent on it before the physical examination.

Examination
This can be subdivided into long or short depending on the history. When examining a joint look at it first. Significant swelling will be immediately apparent and deformity (such as patella dislocation) should not be missed. The step deformity of the subluxed or dislocated acromioclavicular joint should be obvious, as would be the more subtle sharpening of the point of the shoulder when that joint is dislocated.

Next feel the joint. The first thing you are going to feel for is the tenderness that is the marker of localised injury. Look at patients' faces for apprehension when you first touch them because once you have hurt them you are going to lose their cooperation.

It is essential to feel the landmark points around a particular joint. Using the ankle as an example, gentle but specific palpation over the swollen lateral structures will separate out the tenderness

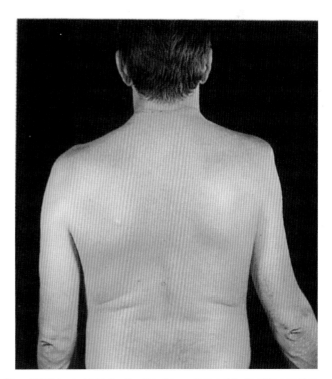

Figure 3.2 Dislocated right shoulder. Note the prominence of the tip of the acromium with a dent below it, rather than a normal deltoid profile

of the fibula itself where it is fractured, from the tenderness overlying the anterior component of the lateral ligament, which runs almost horizontally forward from the tip of the fibula and is far more frequently injured. In the knee, it is very important to remember that the lower end of the medial collateral ligament inserts some 10 cm below the joint line and if you do not feel here you are going to miss sprains of this structure. Bone contours can be palpated and this is particularly useful at the elbow where the loss of the triangular relationship between the olecranon and the medial and lateral epicondyles is an indicator of a dislocation. At the shoulder, the relationship between the front of the humeral head and the coracoid process is altered in dislocations and there is a palpable step deformity in significant lesions of the sterno-clavicular joint.

Now move the joint. There is no need to assess much active movement other than to establish whether or not the joint can move. In this early stage, pain will inhibit so much movement that anything more than the most simple active movement is not really helpful. Lack of movement will detect lesions such as a tear of the extensor apparatus of the knee, but a tear of the rotator cuff in the shoulder or even a tear of the Achilles tendon may be disguised by the activity of muscles, such as deltoid or flexor hallucis longus.

I find passive range of motion to be more helpful. Where passive movement is restricted, it is necessary to decide whether this is because of pain from muscle spasm, because the joint itself is not in the normal position (dislocated), or because something within the joint is blocking the movement (locked knee, which inter alia, means lack of full extension). You are, to some extent, dependent upon how soon after the acute injury you see the patient. If you are a club doctor on the touchline, then often you will be able to assess the joint before the painful muscle spasm has set in and stopped it moving. You may well have the benefit over a subsequent examiner. For the next few days it is very difficult to distinguish between these three things and it may well only be in the fortnight or so after the injury that it becomes possible again to separate out these categories.

Look for **abnormal** movement of the joint. Using the knee as an example, is there abnormal opening of the inner or outer side when you apply a stress. In this particular joint, remember that the posterior structures (less frequently injured) can maintain stability in the fully straightened knee, so you have got to relax those by bending it to about 30° then you can apply a valgus or varus force (while making sure the leg is not rotating) and establish whether the collateral ligaments have been torn. In this same position at about 30°, you can stabilise the femur in one hand and gently pull the tibia forward. This is perhaps the easiest test of the integrity of the anterior cruciate ligament. When positive, the tibia moves forward more than the other side and there is no firm "end point". This is the Lachman test.

Investigation

If the patient is in the surgery and has an acutely swollen joint (usually the knee), aspirate it. Is there blood in the joint? The message in the knee is that 75% or so of acute haemarthroses are caused by a torn anterior cruciate. The technique is simple; with clean hands simply clean the skin with standard solution, then introduce a light blue needle above the superolateral aspect of the patella through all the structures pointing to the back of the mid point of the patella. This will enter the joint and you can then aspirate. This is not a therapeutic aspiration; you need to get a cubic centimetre or so into the syringe just to be sure that it is a genuine haemarthrosis and not a little blood from the perforated soft tissues. It is often easy to remove a lot more, and this makes the joint far more comfortable.

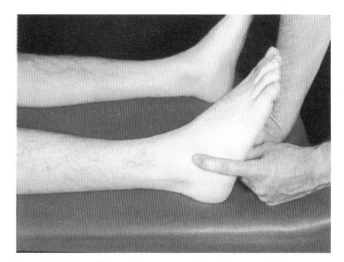

Figure 3.3 Palpation of the anterior component of lateral ligament of ankle

---

Stages before reaching diagnoses

- History of how the injury was sustained
- Examination:
  Look for swelling, bruising, skin lesions, bone deformity
  Feel for tenderness (bone or ligament), bone contours, relations between bones, or deformity
  Move the joint (check particularly for passive and abnormal movement
- Investigations:
  Aspiration for blood (haemarthrosis)
  Radiology (plain, ultrasound scanning)
- Diagnosis
  Differential and *favoured*

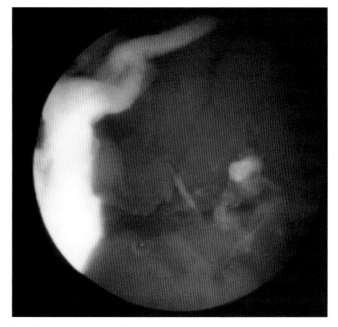

Figure 3.4 Arthroscopic view of blood in a joint — haemarthrosis

In twenty years, I have never seen subsequent infection in a joint of a patient who did not have some risk factor, such as immunosuppression, diabetes, or a skin lesion at the site of the needle puncture.

With a syringe full of blood you know this patient must be urgently evaluated elsewhere, but draw some air into the syringe and rotate it to coat the walls with the blood. If there are any fat globules in the film there is an intra-articular fracture as well.

The usual special investigation is an X-ray. After physical examination, the doctor must give the radiologist a history and differential diagnosis. Only in this way can a sensible report be provided (and the appropriate part to be X-rayed). For example, without examination of the injured wrist, X-rays of this joint rather than scaphoid views will be requested. An X-ray of the leg will usually show the ankle. The picture has not been centred for that joint and most fine detail will not be possible. You must examine the joint and be specific about what you want X-rayed.

There are other investigations that may be done, such as bone scans, CT scans and MRI, but they usually follow hospital referral.

Diagnosis

By now there should be a differential diagnosis, with a favoured diagnosis. It is always slightly consoling that a relatively small number of things can happen to a joint and its surrounding structures.

Skin

In reviewing the joint from the outside, start from the skin. Impacts over joints are frequent and hard grounds or artificial surfaces create significant skin lesions, caused by shear forces. Such lesions may also be indicators of the underlying joint problem. In all cases these need to be cleaned and covered with a breathing adhesive drape that allows protected rapid healing.

Muscles

More deeply sited are contusions in and around muscles. These may produce very spectacular results indeed. The intermuscular haematoma may produce its bruising along the whole length of the limb simply because the blood tracks between the muscle bellies and may pop to the surface almost anywhere. Although a bit sore, movement of the joint either remains full or rapidly returns to normal. Intramuscular haematoma is where the bleeding is contained within the muscle sheath. Pressures here can become quite high and this type of injury produces very profound stiffness that may be slow to resolve. In all contusions of this nature, the old standards of rest, ice, compression, and elevation cannot be bettered. The main risk is that of myositis ossificans. This is a condition in which the injured muscle starts calcifying and laying down a bone-like substance. There is extreme stiffness. There may be an associated joint effusion. Aggressive mobilisation makes it worse and indomethacin is the treatment of choice. Rest the limb of the injured joint and encourage or allow the athlete to use the uninjured limbs (the other three corners) and to maintain cardiovascular status. Rest applies to the joint not the patient. Ice (although poorly understood) is hallowed by tradition and seems to be effective. It should be wrapped in a towel and not applied directly to the skin. A traditional source of this appropriate low temperature material is a bag of frozen peas straight from the freezer (wrapped in a cloth to stop burning). Compression for most people is use of a crepe bandage, but equipment capable of pulsing compression, such as the aircast system, is more widely used. The whole aim of the compression is to reduce the volume of the inflammatory fluid and enable the cells to restore normality without laying down fibrous tissue as this, inevitably, leads to stiffness. Elevation is

Causes of haemarthrosis
• Torn anterior cruciate ligament (in 75%) • Meniscus tear • Chondral separation

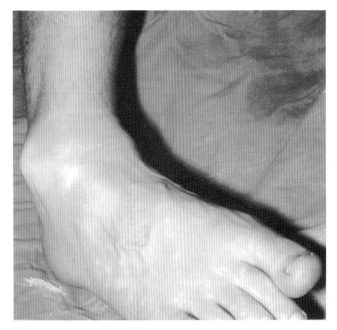

Figure 3.5 Ankle dislocation with skin at risk over the lateral malleolus

Muscle injuries

• Intermuscular haematomas
  Bruising (full length of limb), slight soreness, movement not (or only briefly) affected
• Intramuscular haematomas
  Profound long-lasting stiffness
  Treatment regimen RICE (rest, ice, compression, and elevation)
• Strain
  To prevent the 'second injury syndrome', ensure that the lesion has healed before sport is started again

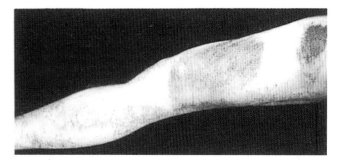

Figure 3.6 Intermuscular haematoma after a kick during a game of rugby

simply another way of achieving the same thing. The patient must be encouraged to move the joint in the inner, pain-free range to maintain mobility and promote healing.

Muscles can also be strained, that is, have a degree of longitudinal failure, usually graded from 1 to 3 where 3 is a complete tear. Hamstring injury is typical; the muscle crosses two joints (the hip and knee) and commonly causes problems with coordination, leading to just a tweak or full disruption. It is frequently forgotten how much muscles protect ligaments. Ligaments of major joints are relatively weak and depend on muscle control for their integrity. If the joint is heavily stressed before those muscles are in control, the ligaments can be injured. This is frequently seen after injury to the quadriceps when the player goes back too soon and tears the ligaments in the knee "second injury syndrome". **Full muscle rehabilitation is essential before return to competition**.

Ligaments

Ligaments are also subject to sprains. These are usually graded into three degrees. A grade I simply has some local tenderness over the ligament, but there is no overt loss of integrity and it is just sore. The treatment is to explain what is happening to the patient. Nonsteroidal anti-inflammatories help to reduce the pain, and mobilisation (with an appropriate support such as a tubigrip) is encouraged.

Grade II reveals a jog of abnormal motion. This means there is still overall integrity of the ligament, but enough has been torn for it to stretch. It, therefore, needs more protection and is a perfect indication for the aircast system, ice, and nonsteroidals. This injury may be seen more commonly around the ankle where the anterior fasciculus of the lateral ligament frequently suffers a grade II injury. Early aggressive treatment in the middle range of movement with compression, elevation, and analgesia produces much better healing than plaster immobilisation, which often leads to failure of proprioception and a so-called chronically unstable joint. Similar injuries are seen at the medial ligament of the knee and a bracing system is very effective, especially by blocking the last few degrees of extension in the early phase of rehabilitation.

Grade III shows major abnormal motion. This must be referred to hospital for accurate assessment possibly under anaesthesia.

Joints

Subluxations

Subluxations are incomplete dislocations where there remains some degree of contact between the articular surfaces. Perhaps the most common example of this is the lesion of acromioclavicular joint. The mechanism is some disruption of the capsule, but the main ligamentous structures have remained intact. There are very few regular contact sportsmen who have not had this injury. It is typified by a slight step deformity and does not require surgery. Subluxations need to be distinguished from dislocations.

Dislocations

Dislocations imply complete loss of contact between the joint surfaces. Continuing with the acromioclavicular analogy, this is a far more important injury. The actual direction of the displacement is not upwards, but backwards and is best detected by accurate observation from above the seated patient.

The most common dislocations are seen at the fingers, shoulder, patella, and elbow. Both the shoulder and elbow may be a little difficult to recognise immediately from observation, but the

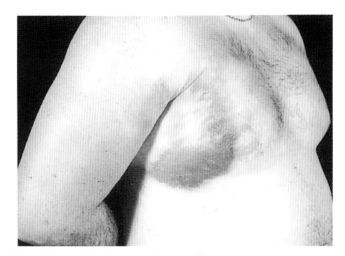
Figure 3.7 Intramuscular haematoma in a power lifter

Sprains of ligaments

- Grade I (local tenderness, normal joint movement)
  Give NSAIDs; support sprain; encourage mobilisation
- Grade II (slightly abnormal joint movement)
  Give more protection, compression, and NSAIDs; raise affected limb; encourage middle range of movement (do not immobilise in plaster
- Grade III (major abnormal joint movement)
  Refer to hospital; possibly examine under anaesthesia

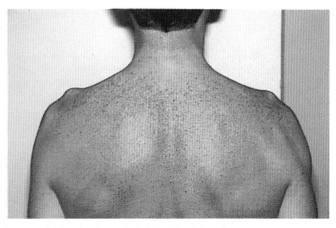
Figure 3.8 Subluxation of acromioclavicular joints (bilateral)

fingers and patella should be obvious. Careful palpation should reveal dislocations at other sites.

Depending on the skill and experience of the doctor, and how quickly after the injury the dislocation is seen, it may be reasonable to attempt immediate reduction. This may, in fact, be easier in cases of recurrent dislocation (usually of the shoulder), but must only be performed in the absence of any complicating factors. These would include any evidence of neurological damage; it is mandatory to be sure that the circumflex nerve is working before reducing a dislocated shoulder. The neuro-vascular status must be checked and recorded post-reduction. Rarely, a fracture dislocation of the ankle may press so hard on the skin that immediate reduction is essential to prevent the skin dying. Once any reduction has been performed, it is essential to have an X-ray, both to confirm the reduction and exclude any associated fractures, even if there has been a pre-reduction film.

Most dislocations can subsequently be safely mobilised within the middle range, protecting the torn structures from the extremes of movement while promoting better healing. Finger dislocations are strapped to the adjacent finger or a double-barrelled finger-sized tubigrip is used and early return to sport is allowed. The dislocated shoulder must be protected until adequate healing has taken place and exercises to build up the muscles on the front of the joint are essential.

Special situations

The immature skeleton
Ligaments are stronger than the epiphysis. In the apparently unstable knee of the child, the movement is often taking place at the distal femoral epiphysis. Stress X-rays must be done. The most common example of this injury is the 'lateral ligament ankle sprain' where the lateral fibular epiphysis has given way, but has sprung back into position. This can be detected by careful palpation and the tenderness will be found exactly over the epiphyseal line of the fibula rather than in the ligaments themselves. This is perhaps one of the few indications for plaster immobilisation of "soft tissue" ankle injury.

Haemarthrosis of the knee
The importance of this injury is not well recognised. The history is usually of a non contact twisting injury of the knee, often associated with an audible crack and followed quickly by swelling. The X-rays of these joints are, with minor exceptions, normal. The rapid swelling indicates a haemarthrosis until proven otherwise. Seventy-five percent of these patients will have a torn anterior cruciate ligament. Of the other causes of bleeding, the majority will be meniscus tear. As the meniscus has bled, it has a blood supply and, if relocated and fixed (a quick and simple procedure through the arthroscope), there is a good chance of it healing. A minority have sustained a chondral separation. This can be relocated and simply fixed, which is essential to avoid exposed bone (osteoarthritis) in a young patient.

In summary, take time to make a diagnosis; this might take a few minutes, but will help your patients and keep you out of the courts.

Once you have established that the neuro vascular status of the limb distal to the injured joint is not compromised, you will not be criticised for supporting and resting the injured joint while seeking more experienced help.

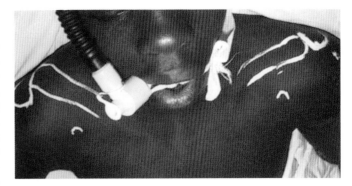
Figure 3.9 Marking to show dislocation of the acromioclavicular joint

Reduction of dislocation or fracture
- Only if there are no complications (for example, neurological damage)
- Easier in recurrent dislocation
- Essential if a fracture causes pressure on skin
- Perform radiography afterwards to rule out fracture and (if there is no fracture, merely dislocation) to check whether reduction has been achieved
- Limit mobility and protect to help joint heal

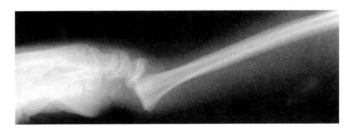
Figure 3.10 Complete separation of the distal radial epiphysis

Acknowledgements

The photograph showing intermuscular and intramuscular haematomas appear (in black and white) in: Helal B, King J, Grange WJ, eds. *Sports injuries and their treatment*. London: Chapman and Hall, 1987. They are reproduced with the kind permission of the publisher.

4 Musculoskeletal injury in the immature athlete

M F Macnicol

The athletic child faces a number of potential problems if dedicated to competitive sport.

Structural

Because the skeleton is growing rapidly, stretching injury to the musculotendinous units is reasonably common, with pain often felt in relation to hamstrings, the patellofemoral mechanism, and the tibialis posterior tendon. Limb length discrepancy or pelvic width in the maturing girl may also predispose to the 'snapping hip syndrome', usually produced by tenting of the fascia lata over the greater trochanter, or occasionally to the psoas tendon subluxing over the anterior aspect of the hip joint in the gymnast. Tension at the attachment of tendon to bone may produce symptoms at sites, such as the tibial tuberosity (Osgood Schlatter's disease), or at the accessory navicular in the medial arch of the foot. Heel pain, sometimes termed Sever's disease, develops from the compressive loading of the posterior calcaneum and its apophysis as a resultant force is generated by the Achilles tendon and the plantar fascia.

Ironically, intrinsic ligament laxity may also predispose to ligament sprains and articular cartilage injuries, especially when there is concomitant malalignment or torsional abnormality, such as persistent femoral anteversion, genu valgum or varum, and pronation (flattening) of the feet. This imbalance between excessive "active" tension and inherent "passive" flexibility produces symptoms, particularly in sports where flexibility is essential.

A final, important structural factor is the presence of the growth plate or physis. This can be injured by repetitive impaction over a prolonged period of time, or by rotational stress (*Figure 4.1*). There is no convincing evidence that long-term, strenuous sporting activity or heavy labour stunts growth in the elongating skeleton, but a variety of injuries will produce partial or complete growth plate arrest. The most common injury that causes a bony tether at the growth plate is fracture (*Figure 4.2*), and approximately 15% of all paediatric fractures involve the growth plate.

Fortunately, the vast majority of fractures do not lead to growth disturbance, but in the type III and IV (Salter Harris) fracture pattern, and in the longitudinal compression type V fracture, growth plate arrest may occur (*Figure 4.3*). It is also occasionally seen after severely displaced type II epiphyseal plate injuries, particularly those involving the distal femur, and in open fracture where the perichondrial ring of the growth plate is damaged.

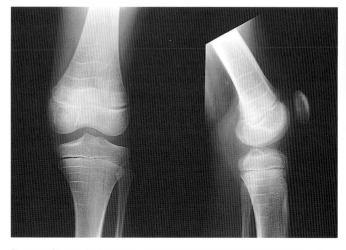

Figure 4.1 Repeated skiing trauma every winter has produced a "ladder" of temporary growth arrest lines in the femur and tibia

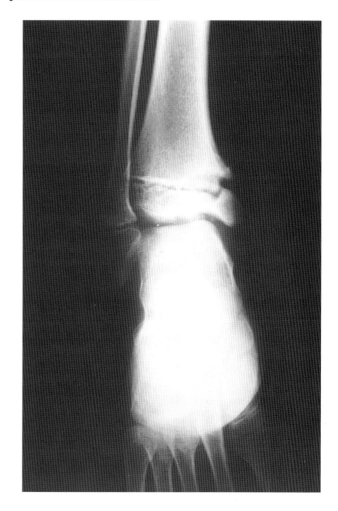

Figure 4.2 Partial growth arrest produced by a splitting (type III) fracture of the distal tibial growth plate from a soccer tackle

Stress fractures are rare in childhood, but may be seen in the upper third of the tibia posteromedially (*Figure 4.4*), the tibial mid-shaft or the lower fibula, the second metatarsal and the femoral neck or shaft. Differentiation from neoplasia or infection is important and isotope, magnetic resonance, or CT scanning should be considered.

Metabolic

Children take longer to acclimatise to a hot or humid environment and may, therefore, suffer more readily from heat exhaustion, cramps, and dehydration. Their characteristic increased ventilation rate may also cause toxic changes in a polluted environment. Paediatric metabolism is anaerobically inferior to the adult, so that endurance sports may be hazardous, probably secondary to limited phosphofructokinase activity and resultant impairment of glycolysis. Despite this, in submaximal activity children reach a steady state more readily and, in the adolescent, metabolic differences are less significant.

With the exception of asthma, and possibly mild diabetes, children with pre-existing metabolic conditions rarely attain major sporting prowess. However, haemophilia and other haematological conditions, hypertension, and convulsive disorders are sometimes unearthed by the stresses of competitive sport. Children with Down's syndrome and skeletal dysplasias associated with ligament laxity, and those with other structural weaknesses, such as hernia, clearly require appropriate supervision and advice, and the dangers of sport related injury should be frankly discussed with the child and his/her parents.

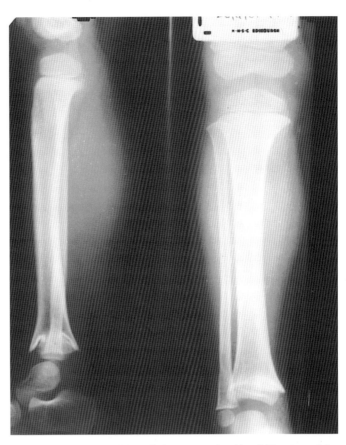

Figure 4.3 Complete distal tibial growth plate arrest produced by a fall from trampolining

Emotional

A child who is gifted athletically may be pressured by competition from his or her peers, or from adults, to perform competitively in a way that ceases to be enjoyable. Some parents live vicariously through the achievements of their offspring and the demands of a gymnastics teacher or coach may exceed the child's interest in a particular sport. This becomes a particular problem during early adolescence when a number of other social and emotional problems are brought to bear. In today's competitive environment, the majority of children cease to undertake sport to any remarkable level of achievement and it is left to a small cohort of physically talented children and adolescents to bear the brunt of ambition, long hours of training, and the highs and lows of competition.

Injury patterns

Sports injuries are rare before the age of eight or nine years, although gymnasts may be an exception to this rule. Progressively, during the later stages of childhood, the athletic individual becomes more prone to musculoskeletal injury. In many instances, the trauma is little different to the child who plays, with abrasions, bruises and haematomas, minor fractures and sprains occurring as a result of falls, collisions, and rotational stresses. Inherent morphological weaknesses, such as patellar instability and spondylolisthesis, become increasingly apparent and various anatomical patterns of injury are seen with different sports.

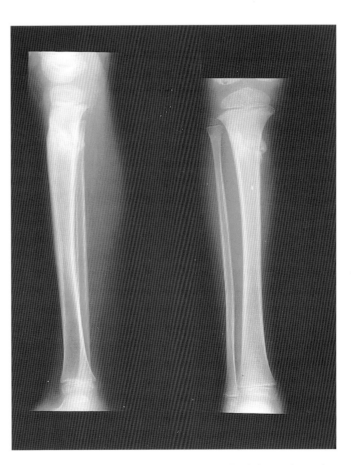

Figure 4.4 A stress fracture at the typical site in the tibia, which is the most commonly affected bone

Head and neck

For example, head injury is more likely as a result of a fall in gymnastics, or from a horse, and is incurred in older children and adolescents from bicycling, diving, and skiing. Contact sports, such as rugby, soccer, and ice hockey, produce a number of facial and head injuries, most of which are relatively trivial. However, boxing carries with it a notorious reputation for cerebral contusion and worse. Children who undertake trampolining, gymnastics, and other sports where falling from a height is likely may also injure the cervical spine. Sprains, fracture dislocations, or subluxations, and vertebral compression injuries represent a small, but severe selection of injuries that are rarely accompanied by neurological deficit in the child.

The arm

The upper limb may be the site of symptoms in children who swim, play racket games or cricket, or who undertake field sports involving throwing. Recurrent dislocation of the shoulder, rotator cuff tears, and later impingement have all been described in the paediatric athlete. Clavicular fractures and subluxations, and occasional nerve compression syndromes are also encountered. The elbow is a common site for fracture, particularly supra-condylar humeral fractures (*Figure 4.5*), and avulsion injuries. Repeated vaulting, or throwing may impart a valgus stress to the elbow, producing impingement at the radiocapitellar region and possibly a chronic ulnar neuritis. Panner's disease of the capitellum is seen before the age of 11 years and, in the adolescent, osteochondritis dissecans, recurrent elbow sub-luxation, and triceps tendinitis (in gymnasts) may be troublesome.

The leg

Lower limb soft tissue injuries are more common than those of the upper limb. When considering the hip joint, it must be remembered that pain could be referred down the anterior obturator nerve to the medial aspect of the knee, confusing the examiner. Dysplasia of the hip and mild deformity secondary to Perthes' disease in mid childhood classically become symptomatic during the later years of childhood or adolescence. Significant slipping of the proximal femoral epiphysis (*Figure 4.6*) is rare, but lesser slipping of both proximal femoral epiphyses is seen in adolescent boys, particularly those who play a great deal of competitive soccer. The minor rotational abnormality of the hip joint then predisposes the individual to later groin strains and eventually, in some cases, to osteoarthritis of the hip. Overuse injuries are as likely to occur in the younger athlete as they are in the adult and consist of submaximal, repetitive stresses that are usually avoidable. In particular, symptoms from a particular form of training should be heeded and the youngster should not be encouraged to "run through" the pain. The snapping hip syndrome mentioned earlier may be a problem in this group, and is seen in gymnasts and dancers. Osteitis pubis and adductor partial tears are occasionally encountered in adolescence, as are stress fractures of the pelvic rim.

More significant avulsion injuries of the pelvis and proximal femur are sometimes encountered (*Figure 4.7*). Usually, these do not require to be openly reduced and fixed, but disability from fibrous union or prominence of an avulsed fragment can be appreciable. Occasionally, the presence of a benign cyst in the femoral neck may lead to femoral neck fracture and subsequent avascular necrosis of the femoral head.

The knee

The knee is a common site of symptomatology with meniscal lesions, such as tears, subluxations, and discoid anomalies increasingly troublesome during mid to late childhood. Wherever

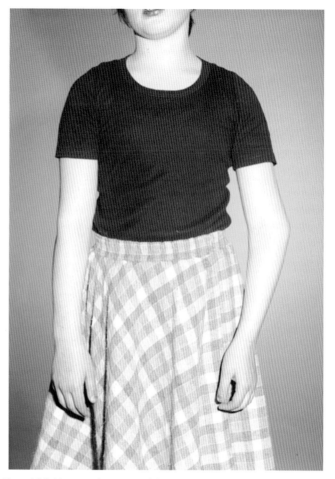

Figure 4.5 Cubitus varus in a gymnast following a supracondyler humeral fracture that was inadequately reduced

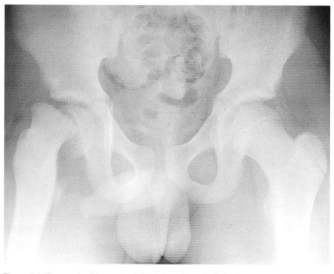

Figure 4.6 The proximal femoral epiphysis has slipped off the femoral neck

possible, peripheral splits of the meniscus through its vascular zone should be allowed to heal, with or without suturing, depending upon the stability of the segment. The advent of the arthroscope and MR scanning has allowed greater precision in diagnosis and treatment, and it is appreciated that the meniscus in childhood is largely vascular and capable of healing. In adolescence, the vascular "front2 recedes from the central portion of the meniscus so that, eventually, much of the meniscus is nourished by synovial fluid rather than by blood vessels.

Patellofemoral pain is a very common concern in childhood and adolescence. The causes may be obvious, but are often not. It is generally accepted that patellar pain is self-limiting and that physiotherapy and an avoidance of certain sports is the logical approach to a common problem. Patellar subluxation should also be treated conservatively if at all possible, since this often becomes less troublesome when skeletal growth has ceased.

Osteochondritis dissecans develops in association with patellar subluxations or impaction injuries between the tibia and the femur. Healing is more certain in the child under the age of 12 or 13 years and in adolescence, separation of an osteochondritic fragment may be better treated by excision of the fragment rather than its replacement and fixation. Early recognition of osteochondritis dissecans is important, so that sport can be reduced and the chance of healing increased.

Significant ligament tears can occur in the younger child, and it is appreciated that cruciate injuries are relatively common in adolescence. Fortunately, in many cases avulsion of the anterior cruciate ligament from the intercondylar eminence makes fixation relatively simple (*Figure 4.8*), although concomitant stretching of the ligament may leave the knee unstable despite surgical intervention.

Posterior cruciate ligaments are more rare, but can be dealt with appropriately if recognised early, particularly avulsions from the posterior proximal tibia.

Autogenous reconstruction of the anterior cruciate ligament is increasingly practised, generally using the hamstring tendons through drill holes in the tibia and the femur. This technique appears to be safe provided that the growth plate has no more than two or three years of activity within it. There remains, however, a risk that the knee may develop hyperextension due to tethering from the tendon graft.

In addition to Osgood Schlatter's disease at the tibial tuberosity, acute fracture of the tibial tubercle may occur, as may sleeve fractures of the lower patella, or the more chronic condition of Sinding-Larsen-Johansson syndrome. These are more likely in children and adolescents with patella alta and instability of the patellofemoral mechanism.

Shin and foot

Stress fractures and tibialis posterior tendinitis ("junior leg") affect the lower leg in runners. Isotope bone scanning is a useful means of identifying a stress fracture, before it becomes radiographically evident, and the third cause of "shin splints" is compartment syndrome which may affect the tibialis anterior and toe extensor muscles in the adolescent. Achilles tendinitis is also encountered in the teenager and, in most of these conditions, a conservative approach is effective.

Sports injuries of the hand and the foot are relatively rare, but heel pain has already been mentioned and children may develop stress fractures of the metatarsal or sesamoid under the great toe, and plantar fasciitis during adolescence. These injuries are seen in basketball and racket sports, and also in dancers. The younger child may develop mid foot pain from Kohler's disease of the navicular, although this is not strictly speaking a sports injury. Similarly, Freiberg's infraction of the second metatarsal may cause

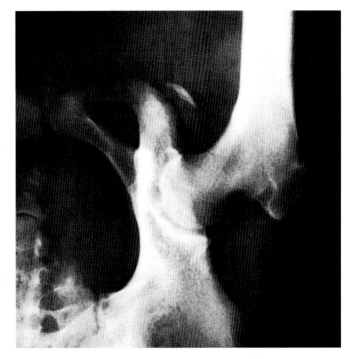

Figure 4.7 Ischial tuberosity avulsion in a rugby player, an injury that mimics a harmstring tear but which should always be suspected in the adolescent

Anterior (patellofemoral) knee pain

Site	Pathology
Patellar	Subluxation
	Compression
	Chondromalacia
	Osteochondritis dissecans
	Osteochondral fracture
	Juvenile chronic arthropathy
Peripatellar	Synovial fringe lesion
	Plica syndrome
	Fat pad pathology
Quadriceps mechanism	Sinding-Larsen-Johansson syndrome
	Patellar tendinitis
	Osgood-Schlatter's disease
	Bursitis
	Cyst
Other	Referred pain — meniscal tear
	— ligament laxity
	— hip pathalogy
	— lumbar nerve
	— root irritation
	Psychosomatic disorder

considerable problems in the teenage girl who enjoys dancing or running. Ankle sprains, principally involving the anterior tibiofibular ligament, are more likely in girls than boys and, as with the cruciate ligaments, may be characterised by bone avulsion rather than an interstitial ligament tear.

Summary

Soft tissue and skeletal injuries are regularly encountered in the sporting child and adolescent. Responsible supervision, an avoidance of significant mismatching in the size of competitors, and education about the nature and treatment of these injuries should lead to less morbidity and parental anxiety.

References

Devas MB (1963) Stress fractures in children. *J Bone Joint Surg* (Br) **45B**: 528–41

Wotten JR, Cross MJ, Holt KW (1990) Avulsion of the ischial apophysis. The case for open reduction and internal fixation. *J Bone Joint Surg* (Br) **72B**: 625–7

Further reading

Sullivan JA, Grana WA, eds (1989) *The Pediatric Athlete*. American Academy of Orthopaedic Surgeons, Illinois

Macnicol MF (1998) *The Problem Knee*, 2nd edn. Butterworth Heinemann, London

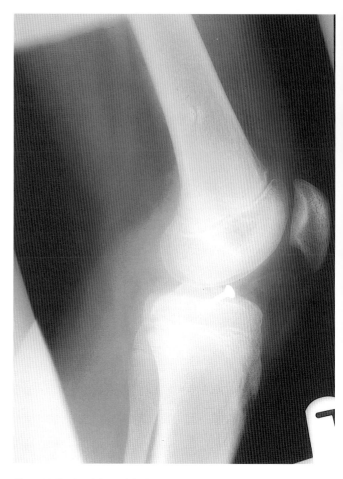

Figure 4.8 Fixation of the avulsed tibial attachment of the anterior cruciate ligament

5 Infections

Geoffrey Pasvol

Competitive sport requires peak performance and even minor physical or psychological injury can blunt achievement. A number of factors predispose sportspeople to infection, such as reduced immunity resulting from stress and overtraining, close contact with others, trauma — especially of the skin, foreign travel, and sexual activity with its concomitant risks of diseases, such as hepatitis B and HIV infection.

Upper respiratory tract infections

Upper respiratory tract infections are of concern to the athlete, especially when recurrent. They are commonly due to viruses, such as enteroviruses (echovirus and coxsackie), adenoviruses and influenza, and β-haemolytic streptococci (*Figure 5.1*). *Chlamydia pneumoniae* has gained notoriety in Swedish orienteers leading to a myocarditis. There are rapid methods available to distinguish these conditions from one another, such as throat culture for β-haemolytic streptococci or a heterophile antibody (Paul-Bunnell) test for infectious mononucleosis. Viral culture and serology in diagnosis is seldom helpful.

Symptomatic relief using analgesics, antihistamines, or decongestants may help in some cases. Group A β-haemolytic streptococcal sore throat is treated with penicillin, or a second generation cefalosporin or erythromycin in the case of penicillin allergy. Treatment should continue for at least ten days to avoid recurrence.

Routes of spread

The young sportsperson is most susceptible to those infections spread by:

	Examples
Droplets	Upper respiratory tract infections
The orofaecal route	Traveller's diarrhoea, hepatitis A and E
Water	Leptospirosis
Direct contact	*Herpes simplex*, impetigo
Wound infection	Tetanus, streptococcal/staphylococcal
Sexual activity	Hepatitis B, HIV
Insect vectors	Malaria, Lyme disease

Whether or not an individual with an upper respiratory tract infection should refrain from exercise is a major issue. In the presence of fever, tachycardia at rest, or severe myalgia or lethargy, athletes should not participate in sport. Complications, such as cardiac arrhythmias, have been overemphasised. Viral myocarditis is a rare event. Sudden cardiac death is more

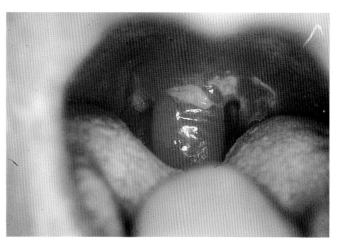

Figure 5.1 Pharyngitis due to the β-haemolytic streptococcus with ulceration of the uvula

---

Some common clinical presentations of EBV infection

- A sore throat with fever and generalised lymphadenopathy (*Figure 5.2*) with or without an enlarged spleen
- In a minority of cases, a diffuse maculopapular rash may be present
- Patients may present with a hepatic illness with jaundice
- A haematological disorder (e.g., thrombocytopenia, haemolytic anaemia or pancytopenia)
- Any neurological disorder ranging from an encephalitis to a peripheral neuropathy.

Complications

There are three complications of EBV infection of particular relevance to athletes:

- **Splenic rupture**: up to 40% of cases of traumatic splenic rupture have occurred in athletes who have, or have subsequently been found to have, infectious mononucleosis
- **Persistent fatigue**: in a minority of cases, fatigue and lethargy may persist for an indefinite period. These cases may include a proportion of individuals with the chronic fatigue syndrome
- **Myocarditis** with a persistent tachycardia, an abnormal ECG, and raised cardiac enzymes

commonly due to hypertrophic cardiomyopathy or undetected coronary artery disease.

The glandular fevers include infectious mononucleosis (due to the Epstein-Barr virus (EBV)), toxoplasmosis, cytomegalovirus infection and, more recently, an HIV seroconversion illness.

Infectious mononucleosis

Infectious mononucleosis (IMN) due to EBV is an important and common infection in athletes. Spread is mainly via intimate close contact; thus isolation of proven or suspected cases is unnecessary. The diagnosis of IMN is made on the basis of a significant number of atypical lymphocytes (>15%) on the peripheral blood film. A heterophile antibody test for IMN, such as the Monospot® test, may be negative in the first week or two of illness and remains negative throughout in about 15% of cases. The serum may also be tested for antibodies against the viral capsid antigen (VCA). A positive VCA IgG test (whatever the titre) in the absence of a positive IgM, indicates only past infection. IMN lasts for about two to six weeks and is self-limiting.

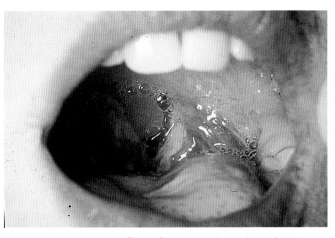

Figure 5.2 Pharyngitis due to the Epstein-Barr virus showing a pale membrane

Treatment

The use of corticosteroids in IMN has only been established in the case of obstructive pharyngitis, whereas the usefulness of corticosteroids in cases with liver, neurological, or haematological involvement is unproven. Corticosteroids have not been shown to reduce the risk of splenic rupture or fatigue. Return to sporting activity after IMN should always be graded and limited to the exercise tolerance of the patient. Total bed rest is unnecessary and may even delay recovery. Since the risk of splenic rupture is greatest in the first months, strenuous exercise and alcohol consumption should be avoided during this period, especially in those undertaking contact sports.

Toxoplasmosis

Toxoplasma gondii, an intracellular protozoan infection acquired from cats and undercooked or raw meat, may produce a glandular fever syndrome with fever, hepatosplenomegaly, and generalised or localised lymphadenopathy. The clinical diagnosis of toxoplasmosis can be confirmed by serology and a fourfold rise or fall in the toxoplasma latex test, or a positive toxoplasma IgM, regardless of titre, is indicative of recent infection. Most episodes of toxoplasmosis are self-limiting and do not require specific treatment in the non-immunocompromised.

Cytomegalovirus

Glandular fever syndrome with or without jaundice due to cytomegalovirus is uncommon and usually self-limiting.

Hepatitis

Sportspeople are particulary prone to hepatitis.

Hepatitis A

Nausea, loss of appetite, vomiting, and abdominal pain in hepatitis A often precede the appearance of jaundice by a number of days and it is during this period that the individual is most infectious. The urine becomes dark due to the presence of bilirubin and the stools light due to intrahepatic cholestasis. Jaundice may then appear and remain for a few days or weeks, followed by a variable period to complete recovery. Hepatitis A is contagious and spreads rapidly. Close contacts should be given passive protection with 250 mg intramuscular gammaglobulin. However, by the time jaundice appears, the need to isolate the patient has passed. The diagnosis is confirmed in the laboratory

More common causes of hepatitis in man

Organism	Transmission route
Hepatitis A virus	Orofaecal
Hepatitis B virus	Blood or sexual contact
Hepatitis C virus	Blood; sexual contact not common
Hepatitis D virus	Only in the presence of hepatitis B virus
Hepatitis E virus	Orofaecal
Less Common	
Epstein-Barr virus	Close contact
Cytomegalovirus	Close contact, blood
Toxoplasma gondii	Contact with cats, undercooked meat
Leptospira spp.	Water

with a hepatitis A virus IgM antibody test. The illness can be monitored by the measurement of liver function tests, such as the transaminases and lactate dehydrogenase, but these do not necessarily correlate with the severity of disease or outcome. Hepatitis A virus IgG indicates past infection only.

Rest is indicated until the symptoms have subsided, but there is no need to wait until liver function tests have returned to normal.

Hepatitis B

The prodromal symptoms are similar to hepatitis A virus infection, but occasionally there may be a preceding skin rash and/or arthralgia. Treatment of acute cases is symptomatic and over 90% recover spontaneously. Careful follow-up of patients with hepatitis B virus infection is important to ensure that they do not develop any of the important sequelae of infection. There is, at present, no indication that chronic carriers of hepatitis B virus should be prevented from participation in sport, except in close contact sports, such as boxing, wrestling, and rugby.

Chronic (post infection) fatigue syndrome

See *Chapter 7*.

Infections of the skin

The skin is one of the main barriers to infection, which is common in sportspeople.

Tetanus

Although rare, tetanus can be fatal and it is essential that all sportspeople who are vulnerable to "dirty" wounds should ensure that their immunisation status is up-to-date. Infection is the result of infection by the organism *Clostridium tetani*. All wounds require careful consideration of whether a booster vaccination, human tetanus immunoglobulin and/or an antibiotic is indicated. Prophylaxis booster vaccination is required:

- if the last immunisation was more than ten years previously
- where the injured did not receive a full course of vaccination
- if the wound involves an appreciable amount of devitalised tissue
- if the wound is a penetrating wound
- where contact with soil or manure is evident
- in the presence of sepsis.

Viral infections

Molluscum contagiosum
Molluscum contagiosum is due to a pox virus. The lesions are recognised by their characteristic umbilicated appearance (*Figure 5.3*). A number of strategies are available for treatment of molluscum: liquid nitrogen can be used locally on the lesions to good effect; an orange stick may be used to release the cheesey material from the lesion; podophylline 25% can be applied to the lesions once or twice weekly.

Herpes simplex
In sports where there is close contact, for example, in rugby and wrestling, it is possible for an individual who is herpetic to transmit the virus to a team mate or to the opposition, leading to herpes gladiatorum or "scrumpox" (*Figure 5.4*). Lesions on the fingers (herpetic whitlow) may be especially painful. Primary herpetic infections may give rise to a high fever, malaise, and prostration. Recurrences generally produce only a local problem with characteristic clustered vesicles on an erythematous base. Herpes simplex infections may occasionally trigger more generalised erythema multiforme type lesions and, sometimes, full blown Stevens-Johnson syndrome with mucous membrane involvement. The primary infection can be treated with an oral antiviral drug, such as valiciclovir or famciclovir. In severe cases, antivirals can be given parenterally.

Warts (verrucas)
Warts due to papova group of viruses may be a particular nuisance if they occur at important sites that interfere with sport. Warts will often disappear without treatment. Wart paints may be useful; a number contain salicyclic acid. Liquid nitrogen may be used in cryotherapy for warts and particularly troublesome warts can be curetted or removed surgically.

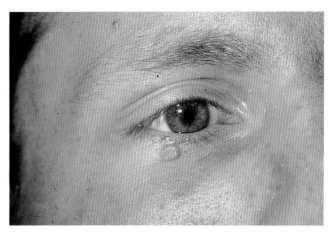
Figure 5.3 Raised pearly-pink lesions of molluscum contagiosum

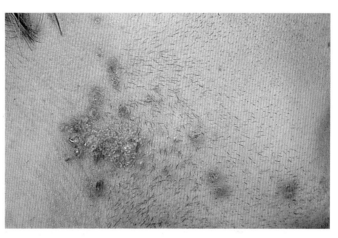
Figure 5.4 Small vesicular lesions of herpes gladiatorum in a rugby player

Bacterial infections

Streptococcal and staphylococcal
Streptococcal and staphylococcal infections of the skin are especially common in athletes. When the lower limb is involved, the portal of entry in sportspeople is often due to athlete's foot. The diagnosis of a streptococcal or staphylococcal skin lesion is most often clinical (*Figure 5.5*). Wound swabs and blood culture may be of help.

Streptococcal or staphylococcal infections may often spread rapidly and need to be urgently treated. The patient needs to be isolated because of easy person-to-person spread. For localised lesions, treatment with oral penicillin and flucloxacillin in combination is usually adequate, although parenteral antibiotics may be required, especially if there are signs of systemic involvement. Systemic involvement is indicated by the clinical state of the patient, for example, a raised temperature, white count, ESR, or C-reactive protein. For patients who are penicillin hypersensitive, a macrolide antibiotic, such as clindamycin, may be used. Meticulous care should be paid to handwashing to avoid local spread of infection.

Recurrent skin and ear infections

Some sportspeople become carriers of staphylococci, which often lead to recurrent infection, especially if the organisms gain access to small cuts and abrasions. Such individuals should pay meticulous care to bathing and, in some cases, may need daily washing with an antiseptic skin cleanser, such as povodine iodine (Betadine®) or chlorhexidine (Hibiscrub®), together with an antibiotic nasal cream containing chlorhexidine (Naseptin®), applied three times a day to the nostril for ten days in order to eradicate carriage of staphylococci.

Otitis externa can be a particular problem in swimmers and is easily diagnosed. The patient has a painful ear with discharge and characteristic erythematous findings on examination of the external auditory meatus. The infecting organisms may be a mixture of gram positive and negative, and treatment may require an antibiotic that is not used topically (such as neomycin or clioquinol). Application of a local cream or ear drops containing an antibiotic and a steroid may be give for seven to ten days.

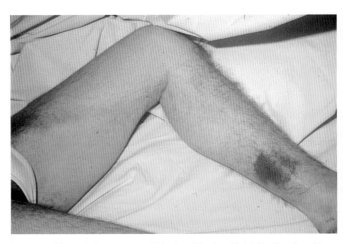

Figure 5.5 β-haemolytic streptococcal infection of the leg with tracking lymphangitis and inguinal lymphadenopathy

Fungal infections

Fungal infections are a particular problem in sites where sweat and moisture accumulate.

Tinea pedis (Athlete's foot)

Athlete's foot characteristically presents as peeling of the skin with fissuring and sometimes secondary infection, especially between the fourth and fifth toes (*Figure 5.6*). It is often associated with blisters on the feet called podopomphylix. The most common infection is due to *Tricophyton rubrum*, although infection due to other fungi also occur. The fissuring may be painful, but the most important complication of Athlete's foot is secondary bacterial infection (ascending lymphangitis and/or cellulitis).

Treatment involves meticulous washing of the feet and careful drying. Application of an antifungal cream, such as cotrimazole, itraconazole or econazole, is effective. Oral terbinafine can be used if the lesions are in an inaccessible site, or are extensive. Nail infections (tinea unguium) can be treated with terbinafine, which produces better results than griseofulvin and requires shorter treatment periods of between six weeks and three months.

Tinea versicolor (Malassezia furfur)

Tinea versicolor produces areas of hypopigmented patches on the skin that are often scaly at the edges (*Figure 5.7*). Treatment consists of the application of selenium sulphide (Selsun®) shampoo. Antifungal imidazole and terbinafine creams are also effective.

HIV infection

The risks of contracting HIV infection in sport related activities must be exceedingly small and to date only one questionable case has been reported. The risk to sportspeople of HIV lies mainly in sexual intercourse. The sharing of razors and tooth brushes has the theoretical possibility of transmitting the virus and should be discouraged. At the same time, it should be emphasised that normal social contact, the sharing of changing facilities, and swimming pools constitute no risk of infection.

In injuries resulting from bleeding of wounds, participants should be aware of the risk and in all cases such wounds should be covered or the player excluded from further participation. All participants, first aid workers and accompanying sports staff

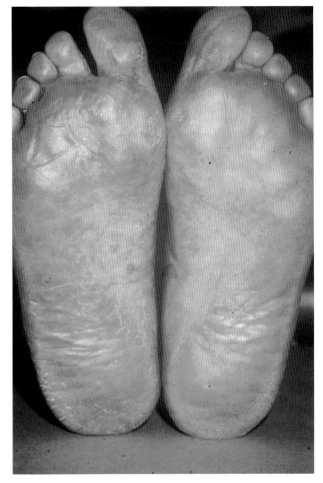

Figure 5.6 Severe involvement of the feet in tinea pedis

Recommendations for handling of injuries on the sportsfield involving sportspersons who may be HIV positive

1   Assume that all casualties are HIV antibody positive

2   Wear gloves for all procedures involving contact with blood or other body secretions

3   Cover all cuts and abrasions where possible

4   Wear protective glasses where blood may be splashed into the face

5   Wash skin immediately after contamination with blood or secretions

6   Dispose of sharps safely: never attempt to resheathe needles

7   Dispose of waste materials by burning

8   Contaminated clothes should be presoaked in hot (>70°C) soapy water for 30 minutes and then washed in a hot cycle washing machine; alternatively, they may be soaked in household bleach (1 in 10 dilution) or Milton® solution for 30 minutes

9   All contaminated equipment or surfaces may be treated with bleach, as above

10   Communal items in the first aid kit no longer have a place in the care of injured sportspeople (for example, bucket and sponge)

11   No cases of HIV infection by mouth-to-mouth resuscitation have been recorded; however, simple devices that prevent direct contact between operator and patient are now available to assist in ventilation

12   Where there has been exposure to blood, further help should be sought with respect to counselling and the need for prophylactic antiviral drugs

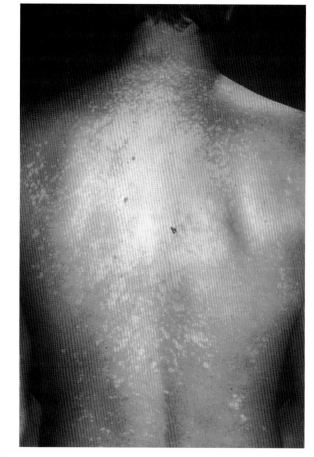

Figure 5.7 Hypopigmentation due to tinea (pityriasis) versicolor

should realise that, other than through sexual contact and other high risk practices, the risks of acquiring HIV infection in sport are very small, but general recommendations may apply.

Travel associated infections

Travellers' diarrhoea

Travellers' diarrhoea is by far the most common illness afflicting travellers and varies with destination. Symptoms most frequently start on the third day abroad. Apart from watery diarrhoea, symptoms include cramps, nausea, vomiting, fever in a few cases, and sometimes frank dysentery. Passage of blood and/or mucus implies bowel inflammation or ulceration and raises the likelihood of an invasive organism, such as *Shigella* species or *Entamoeba histolytica*, although *Salmonella* and *Campylobacter* can produce a similar picture.

Giardiasis has a longer, and often more variable, incubation period (frequently measured in weeks rather than days) and often produces persistent diarrhoea, flatulence, abdominal distension, and lactose intolerance. *Cyclospora* as a cause of travellers' diarrhoea is a recent finding, especially in travellers to Nepal.

Dietary precautions, such as care in selecting well cooked food and consumption of only fresh fruit and vegetables that require peeling, are particularly important. Salads and uncooked shellfish are considered high risk. Only sterilised water should be consumed, including when brushing teeth and for ice in drinks. Because of their low pH (around 5.5) which kills organisms, bottled carbonated drinks are safe. Prophylactic antimicrobials may be indicated in athletes who are staying abroad for less than

Principal causes of travellers' diarrhoea

- Bacteria
  - Enterotoxigenic *Escherichia coli* (ETEC)
  - *Shigella spp.*
  - *Salmonella spp.*
  - *Campylobacter jejuni*
  - *Vibrio cholera*
  - Non-cholera vibrios, for example, *V. parahaemolyticus*
- Viruses
  - Rotavirus
  - Small round viruses, for example, Norwalk agent
- Protozoa
  - *Giardia lamblia*
  - *Entamoeba histolytica*
  - *Cryptosporidium parvum*
  - *Cyclospora cayetanensis*

two weeks and for whom it is vital that peak performance is assured. In this case, the drug of choice would be ciprofloxacin (500 mg, twice daily) since it covers the majority of gut pathogens. Both cotrimoxazole (960 mg, twice daily) or trimethoprim (200 mg, twice daily) for five days have also been shown to be effective. The treatment of travellers' diarrhoea is symptomatic. Milk should be avoided when symptoms are severe. Painful spasms may be treated with co-phenotrope (Lomotil®) or loperamide (Imodium®). These drugs should be used with caution and only for short periods of time, since nausea, vomiting, and sedation are associated with increasing doses, especially in the presence of renal impairment. They should not be used when the diarrhoea is bloody.

Brief guidelines for malarial chemoprophylaxis

The spread of drug-resistant *Plasmodium falciparum* malaria has complicated malarial chemoprophylaxis, as well as the awareness that some of the more effective combination drugs, such as Fansidar®, Maloprim®, and amodiaquine, may have severe and sometimes fatal side effects. Further expert advice may often be required.

Chemo-prophylaxis	Area to be visited	Doses/comments
None	North Africa (Morocco, Algeria, Tunisia, Libya, tourist areas of Egypt); tourist areas of South East Asia (Thailand, Philippines, Hong Kong, Singapore, Bali, China, Vietnam	
Chloroquine or	Middle East (including summer months in rural Egypt and Turkey) Central America, rural Mauritius	300 mg base (2 tablets once per week)
proguanil (Paludrine®)		200 mg once per day
Chloroquine and proguanil	Sub-Saharan Africa, Indian subcontinent, Afghanistan and Iran, South America	Doses as above
Mefloquine (Lariam®)	Sub-Saharan Africa, Papua New Guinea, Solomon Islands and Vanuatu	250 mg (one tablet) once a week. An alternative to chloroquine and proguanil in areas of high risk. Possible increased risk of neuropsychiatric side effects
Doxycycline	Mefloquine-resistant areas of South East Asia (for example. Thai-Cambodian, Thai-Myanmar borders)	100 mg per day

If there is any doubt, specialist advice should be sought. Chemoprophylaxis should start at least a week before departure, continue while away, and for four weeks after return. The possibility of malaria should be considered in any person with a fever who is or has been in a malarious area, whether or not they have been taking antimalarial chemoprophylaxis. At present, no antimalarial can guarantee absolute protection.

Vaccination of travellers

Vaccination of travellers has become a routine but needs to be undertaken with consideration of the risks or benefits involved.

Vaccine	Dose	Comments
Polio	3 drops	Primary course: 3 doses 1 month apart. Boost every 10 years
Tetanus (adsorbed tetanus toxin)	0.5 ml subcutaneously	Primary course: 3 doses 1 month apart. Boost every 10 years up to a maximum of 5 vaccinations unless at special risk
Typhoid		
a) Monovalent typhoid vaccine	0.5 ml intramuscularly for first dose, then 0.2 ml intradermally	Primary course: 2 doses preferably a month and not less than 10 days apart. Boost every 5 years unless at special risk
b) Live oral typhoid* vaccine strain Ty21A	3 enteric coated capsules on alternate days	Boost every 3 years unless at special risk
c) Vi capsular polysaccharide typhoid vaccine	0.5 ml subcutaneously or intramuscularly once only	Single boost every 3 years
Cholera	0.5 ml intramuscularly (first dose), then 0.1 ml intradermally	Primary course: 2 doses preferably a month and not less than 10 days apart. Boosters every 6 months. A poor vaccine
Yellow fever*	0.5 ml subcutaneously	Single injection from a recognised yellow fever centre with certificate (valid 10 days after vaccination for 10 years)
Hepatitis A (human diploid cell)	1 ml intramuscularly	Primary course: a single dose (>1440 ELISA units of hepatitis A protein). For immunity up to 10 years, booster at 6 to 12 months.
Hepatitis B	1 ml intramuscularly	Primary course: 0, 1 and 6 months. 1 booster at 3–5 years
Rabies (human diploid cell vaccine)	1 ml intramuscularly or 0.1 ml intradermally**	Primary course: 3 doses 1 month apart. Booster every 2–3 years

* Indicates live vaccine

** Not standard recommendation, but probably as effective, cheaper and less likely to cause side-effects.

Further reading

Goodman RA, Thacker SB, Solomon SL, Osterholm MT, Hughes JM (1994) Infectious diseases in competitive sports. *JAMA* **271**: 862–67

Mast EE, Goodman RA (1997) Prevention of infectious disease transmission in sports. *Sports Med* **24**: 1–7

Sevier TL (1994) Infectious disease in athletes. *Med Clin N Am* **78**: 389–412

6 Respiratory limitations to aerobic performance in sport

Mark Harries

How muscle leads oxygen demand

Oxygen supply to the muscle is governed by cardiac output, the amount of haemoglobin in circulation and the extent to which haemoglobin is saturated with oxygen (usually greater than 98%). Oxygen demand is driven by the mitochondria, intracellular organelles that contain DNA deriving uniquely from maternal origins and which control the rate at which carbon atoms from glucose and long chain fatty acids are burned with oxygen. During heavy exertion, demand usually outstrips supply. This statement can be made with some confidence because of the unique property of glucose metabolism, which permits the conversion of pyruvate to lactate without the need for additional oxygen. The reaction is fully reversible and once oxygen becomes available again, lactate is reconverted to pyruvate and thence via acetyl Co-enzyme A to the citric acid cycle or back up to glucose. Oxygen consumption rates reach a maximum when the aerobic demands of muscle can no longer be met. The switch to anaerobic metabolism results in lactate spilling from muscle into peripheral blood.

Lactate production may be regarded as a sump into which the glycolytic processes (and hydrogen ions) can be poured without a necessary reduction in activity levels. The extent to which one can continue to "consume one's own smoke" is reflected in the plasma lactate level. Production and consumption rates balance at around 4 mmol/l but levels as high as 20 mmol/l can be tolerated by some athletes over short periods of time with appropriate training. This outlet for fuel consumption is available only to glucose since long chain fatty acids cannot be metabolised without oxygen

Maximal oxygen consumption

Oxygen consumption (VO_2 litres per minute), i.e. aerobic power, is estimated by measuring cardiac output and the arterio–venous oxygen difference. A less invasive method is based upon the assumption that the alveolar capillary membrane is fully permeable to gas and that perfusion matches ventilation. In this case, it is necessary only to know the expired air oxygen fraction and the minute volume. Maximum consumption rates (VO_2 max) in the most highly trained can reach over 90 ml/kg/min or 8l/min absolute (*Figure 6.2*). In sedentary individuals, a 15–20% increase in oxygen consumption may be seen following as little as 3 to 4 weeks hard training, probably due to mitochondrial hypertrophy within the myocytes. There is hot debate as to whether it is the heart or the lungs that ultimately limit exercise performance. However, arterial hypoxaemia seen during heavy exercise (especially in women) suggests that the rate limitation may well lie

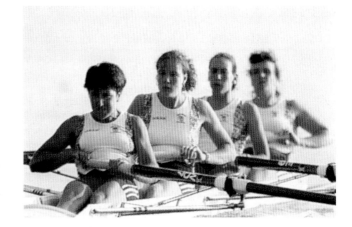

Figure 6.1 Rowing requires high ventilatory capacity

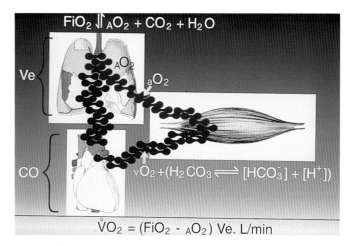

$$VO_2 = (FiO_2 - {}_AO_2)\ Ve.\ L/min$$

Figure 6.2 Directly estimated oxygen consumption (i.e. power output) is the product of cardiac output (CO) and the arterio-venous oxygen difference; $VO_2 = CO\ (aO_2–vO_2)$ l/min. However, assuming gas exchange in the lungs is normal, this figure can be derived from the product of minute ventilation (Ve) and the inspired/expired (alveolar) oxygen difference $VO_2 = Ve\ (FiO_2–{}_AO_2)$ l/min

with gas exchange in the lungs rather than any restriction to cardiac output.

How the lungs may restrict oxygen delivery

Limits to oxygen saturation of haemoglobin

Oxygen is virtually insoluble in plasma, a situation transformed by the presence of haemoglobin, which carries 1.306 ml of oxygen with every gram when fully saturated. Oxygen delivery to tissues is the product of cardiac output, haemoglobin concentration, the oxygen carrying potential of haemoglobin and percentage saturation, not arterial oxygen tension. The s-shaped way in which oxygen dissociates from haemoglobin means that a relatively large fall in arterial oxygen tension, say from 15 kPa to around 8 kPa, can occur without any appreciable change in percentage saturation. This allows terrestrial creatures to function normally through a wide range of altitudes.

Haemoglobin percentage saturation is a reflection of the effectiveness with which air and blood are mixed in the lungs. Normally, perfusion closely matches ventilation and the alveolar capillary membrane is fully permeable to gas. The erythrocytes require only around 0.3 second in the alveolar capillaries to become fully saturated with oxygen. Transit time is normally around 0.8 second and so the erythrocytes should always emerge from the lungs fully saturated with oxygen even during moderately heavy exercise. But in the highly trained at the limits of human performance, transit time can fall below 0.3 second and arterial desaturation may result. The reason that this occurs more readily in young women is unclear but may suggest an additional mismatch of ventilation with perfusion due to the smaller airways of women compared to men. This problem is exacerbated at altitude where the driving pressure across the alveolar capillary membrane is decreased.

Limits to ventilatory capacity

Cardiac output and minute ventilation rise in tandem roughly in the ratio of 1:4. Minute ventilation (Ve 1/min) is the product of breath frequency and tidal volume. Breath frequency at rest averages 15 per minute rising to around 1 per second during high intensity exercise. Since approximately half of the respiratory cycle is expiration, few untrained individuals are able to better a tidal volume that exceeds half of that which they can forcibly expire in 1 second; Ve max 1/min = ½ FEV1 x 60. This represents only around 50% to 80% of what can be achieved by voluntary effort when subjects are asked to breath flat out for 10 seconds (maximum voluntary ventilation, MVV), indicating that, for the untrained at least, the lung should not limit exercise capacity. However, elite performers can exercise for sustained periods at very close to their MVV and, when exercising in their chosen sport, may, occasionally, record higher levels of ventilation than they are able to reach by voluntary effort when at rest.

There is a close relationship between power output (oxygen consumption) and minute ventilation. If, for any reason, minute ventilation is reduced, so, too, is oxygen consumption (*Figure 6.3*). Minute ventilation is restricted largely by the resistance to air flow imparted by the central airways (the peripheral ones less so

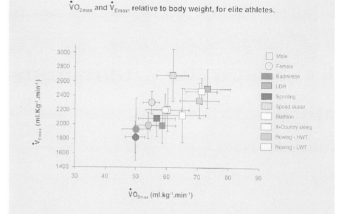

Figure 6.3 Minute ventilation (ml/kg/min) and maximum oxygen consumption measured during maximal exercise in over 600 highly elite male (□) and female (O) athletes attending the British Olympic Medical Centre. The higher the maximal oxygen consumption, the higher also is minute ventilation. The plot for more sedentary individuals will be shifted downwards and to the left. Weight for weight, those with the highest aerobic power are the endurance athletes (for example, marathon runners)

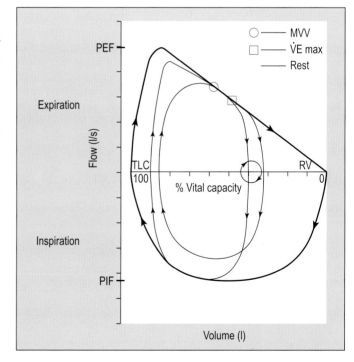

Figure 6.4 The maximum effort flow loop marks out the envelope within which all respiratory efforts are contained. Flow rates have been plotted at tidal breathing, during maximal exercise (VE max) and finally at maximum voluntary ventilation (MVV). The arrows indicate the direction of air flow. The limits of air flow are only reached during expiration while exercising maximally and during both expiration and inspiration at MVV. Notice that as minute ventilation increases, the flow loops are displaced to the left, i.e. towards total lung capacity. In other words, in order to increase minute ventilation the subject must use a higher lung capacity

because there are so many more of them). Change in air flow occurring throughout the respiratory cycle is depicted by the maximum effort flow volume loop. Flow is highest close to total lung capacity (TLC) when the airways are at their widest and lowest at residual volume (RV). The maximum effort flow loop marks out the envelope within which all respiratory efforts are contained; the larger the loop, the greater the minute ventilation that can be achieved and hence the greater the potential power output. Flow rate limitation with increasing exertion is encountered first in expiration and, during MVV, in both expiration and inspiration (*Figure 6.4*).

Asthma limiting ventilatory capacity

To a degree, there is some variability in the shape of the expiratory flow loop between top athletes. One must, therefore, assume that those with lower expiratory flow rates adapt their respiratory efforts in order to perform at the same level as those with higher flows. However, problems arise when there is a sudden detriment in pulmonary function within any one subject, such as occurs in exercise-induced asthma. Here, bronchial narrowing and consequent fall in minute ventilation can have a major effect on aerobic performance with an impact, most significantly, on the endurance sports. Exercise-induced bronchial narrowing is a finding common to all asthmatics, presenting first with a fall in mid expiratory flow (i.e. flow at 50% of vital capacity), then peak expiratory flow rate and finally with a fall in vital capacity. The diagnosis of exercise-induced asthma is established by comparing the shapes of two maximum effort expiratory flow loops, one measured before and a second 10 minutes after a period of vigorous running outdoors lasting 3 to 4 minutes. A fall in mid expiratory flow of greater than 20% after exercise is a positive test (*Figure 6.6*).

Corticosteroids inhaled twice daily are highly effective in blocking exercise-induced bronchial constriction. The dry powders (budesonide, fluticasone, and beclomethasone) have been shown to be more effective than metered dose inhalers. For less severe symptoms, a short-acting β agonist (salbutamol or terbutaline) may be taken 10 minutes before competition. Treatment must be declared to the authorities in advance, stating the diagnosis, medication, and dosage taken. **The medical commission of the International Olympic Committee has ruled that these medications may not be taken in tablet form**.

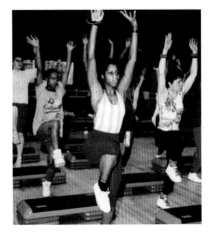

Figure 6.5

Figure 6.6 Exercise-induced asthma can be diagnosed by comparing two static maximum effort flow loops, one measured before (thin line) and another approximately ten minutes after exercise. Flow rate limitation only occurs during expiration and so the inspiratory portion of the loop can be ignored. The earliest indication of asthma is a fall in mid expiratory flow (i.e. flow at 50% of vital capacity); this is followed by a fall in peak expiratory flow and, finally, as symptoms worsen, by a fall in vital capacity as well. The fall in mid expiratory flow of greater than 20% indicates a positive test

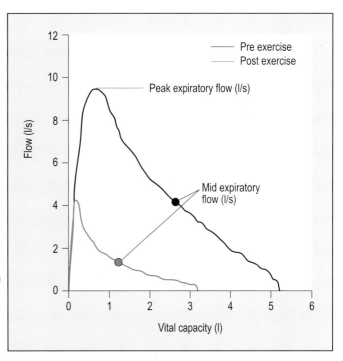

Further reading

Dempsey JA (1986) Is the lung built for exercise? *Med Sci Sports Ex* **18**: 143–55

Harm CA, McClaran S, Nickele GA, Pegelow DF, Nelson WD, Dempsey JA (1998) Exercise-induced aterial hypoxaemia in healthy young women. *J Physiol (Lond)* **507**: 619–28

Whipp BJ, Ward SA (1998) Respiratory responses of athletes to exercise. In: Harries M, Williams C, Stanish WD, Micheli LJ, (eds). *Oxford Textbook of Sports Medicine*, 2 edn. Oxford University Press. Oxford: 17–32

Acknowledgements

I am grateful to Steve Jackson of the British Olympic Medical Centre for his help in preparing *Figure 6.3*.

The photograph of the women's coxless four in the Olympic regatta at Bayolas, Spain, in 1992 was taken by Peter Spurrier, Sports Photography; that of Liz McGolgan in the 10 000 m heats at the Barcelona Olympics in 1992 by Professional Sport; and that of a step aerobics class by Richard J Sowersby.

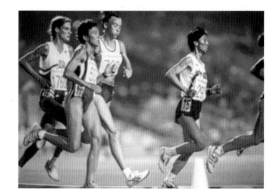

Figure 6.7

7 The overtraining syndrome

Richard Budgett

Athletes may experience chronic fatigue for many reasons, but it often results from a failure to recover from the stress of training and competition—when it is called the overtraining syndrome. The primary complaint is of reduced performance, which is objective and can be measured. Many athletes train at an elite level even to compete domestically, so fatigue due to the stress of training is not confined to Olympic athletes; 10% of college swimmers in the United States are described as burning out each year.

The cause of the overtraining syndrome is not known and there is no diagnostic or warning test. Intensive interval work (high intensity exercise with little rest) is most likely to precipitate the syndrome, so it is extremely rare in sprinters because they train with large amounts of rest. Sprinters may, however, suffer from postviral and other forms of chronic fatigue.

Definitions

Overtraining

Overtraining is the process of excessive training that leads to the overtraining syndrome, which can be defined as a state of prolonged fatigue and underperformance caused by hard training and competition. There should be an objective measure of the loss of form; it should have lasted for at least two weeks, despite adequate rest, and have no identifiable medical cause. Symptoms of a minor infection, typically an upper respiratory tract infection, may recur each time the athlete returns to training after inadequate rest.

Over-reaching

Over-reaching is the process of hard training that enables athletes to reach their full potential. It is part of a planned programme to stimulate adaptation and, when combined with periods of rest, permits the normal physiological response of full supercompensation. This contrasts with the pathological response to training in the overtraining syndrome.

Presentation

Symptoms

Athletes present with fatigue, heavy muscles, underperformance, and depression. Direct questioning reveals poor sleep in over 90% with difficulty getting to sleep, nightmares, waking in the night, and waking unrefreshed. This may be important in the pathogenesis. Other symptoms are: loss of purpose, energy, competitive drive, and libido; emotional lability; increased anxiety and irritability; loss of appetite with weight loss; excessive sweating and a raised resting pulse rate. Some athletes continually catch minor infections every time they build up their training.

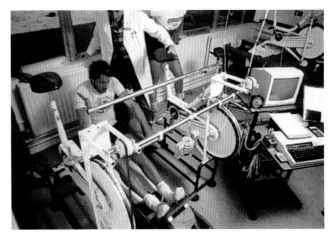

Figure 7.1 Wingate test of upper body in rowers (Steve Redgrave, quadruple Olympic winner)

> **Overtraining**—hard training without adequate rest (pathological)
>
> **Over-reaching**—hard training with adequate rest (normal)

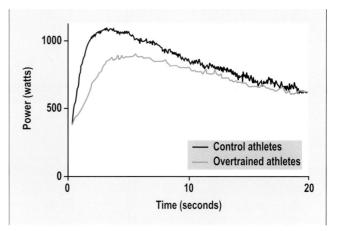

Figure 7.2 Wingate test showing lower peak power in overtrained athletes

Training stresses

The history usually involves an increase or change in training. Many athletes break down when they switch from low intensity winter training to high intensity summer training with intensive interval work. The stress of competition and selection pressures may also contribute. The athletes can usually keep up at the beginning of a race, but describe an inability to lift the pace or sprint for the line.

Inadequate recovery is the vital factor. One swimmer broke the British record and then decided to cut his rest day to train seven days a week instead of six. He broke down after several months and took many weeks to recover. Another swimmer increased his training to eight hours a day; for four months his performance improved, but then he started to fail to recover from training and took months to recover form.

Some suddenly increase their training in order to catch up after a break due to illness or injury when it would be sensible to increase training gradually. They become more desperate and train harder as they fall further behind.

Occasionally training may be heavy, monotonous, and without periodisation (cyclical variation of training). This means that there is no chance to recover, improve, or benefit from exercise.

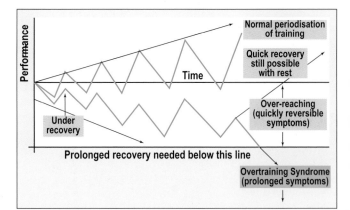

Figure 7.3 Overtraining or under-recovery, leading to the overtraining syndrome

---

Precipitating factors of the overtraining syndrome

- Training
  - intensive interval training
  - sudden increases
  - large volumes of monotonous training
- Stress of competition and selection
  - physical stresses
  - glycogen depletion
  - dehydration
  - other illness or injury
  - psychological stress of life events (for example, moving house, examinations, relationship problems)

Symptoms of overtraining

- Underperformance
- Depression (loss of purpose, competitive drive, and libido)
- Loss of appetite and weight
- Increased anxiety and irritability
- Fatigue
- Sleep disturbance (in over 90% of cases) —difficulty getting to sleep, waking in the night, nightmares, and waking unrefreshed
- Frequent minor infections, particularly of the upper respiratory tract
- Raised resting pulse rate
- Excessive sweating

Other stresses

Stresses, such as examinations and other life events, glycogen depletion, and dehydration will reduce the ability to recover from, or respond to, heavy training. However, it is rare for athletes to break down after less than two weeks of hard training (as in a typical training camp) provided that they then rest and allow themselves to recover afterwards.

Signs

These are inconsistent and generally unhelpful in making the diagnosis. They include increased postural drop in blood pressure and postural rise in heart rate, slow return of the pulse to normal after exercise, decreased lactic acid levels during exercise, reduced maximum oxygen uptake and maximal power output, and increased submaximal oxygen consumption and pulse rate.

Investigation

It is often difficult to persuade athletes and coaches that overtraining has caused underperformance and it is helpful to change the name to 'under-recovery syndrome'. Investigations are needed to exclude other causes of chronic fatigue and to convince an athlete that there is no undiagnosed illness. The range of these tests depends on a sensible approach to clinical possibilities. Serious disease, such as viral myocarditis and arrhythmia, is rare, but must be excluded if suspected. Prolonged glycogen depletion, as in anorexia nervosa, may cause chronic

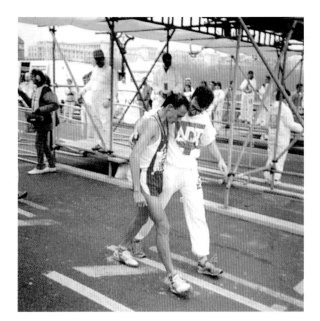

Figure 7.4

fatigue in its own right. A history of recurrent upper respiratory tract infections may represent allergic rhinitis or exercise-induced asthma, in which case lung function tests are needed.

Laboratory tests

Laboratory tests are occasionally helpful but their use in diagnosing and monitoring chronic fatigue in athletes has been over-rated.

Haemoglobin concentrations and packed cell volume

These decrease as a normal response to heavy training. An athlete's reported anaemia is often physiological, due to haemodilution, and does not affect performance. However, increasing the haemoglobin by altitude training or blood doping (cheating) does seem to improve performance.

Ferritin

Low serum ferritin concentrations (reflects low iron stores) can cause fatigue in the absence of anaemia. If the ferritin concentration is very low, treating an athlete with iron by mouth is reasonable.

Creatine kinase

There is a wide individual variation (50-fold) in the response to hard exercise. Serum concentrations above 2000 mmol/l have been seen in normal marathon runners and are not an indication of who will break down with chronic fatigue.

Viruses

Viral titres must be shown to rise and the history is normally suggestive of a post-viral illness. The Paul-Bunnell test is diagnostic and there may be high serum levels of enteroviral particles.

Trace elements and vitamins

There is no proven link of vitamin or trace elements to the overtraining syndrome, and the widespread use of supplements by athletes does not seem to offer any protection from chronic fatigue.

Prevention and early detection

Athletes can tolerate different levels of training and competition stress; overtraining for one may be insufficient training for another. Each athlete's tolerance level will also change through the season, so training must be individualised and varied and should be reduced at times of other stresses, such as exams. Unfortunately, athletes are exhausted most of the time unless they are tapering for a competition, so it is difficult for them to differentiate between overtraining and over-reaching. Investigators have tried to identify strategies for early detection.

In American college swimmers, a 10% incidence of burnout was reduced to zero by daily mood monitoring with a profile of mood state (POMS) questionnaire, and by reducing training when mood deteriorated and increasing it when mood improved.

A persistent rise in early morning heart rate despite rest is non-specific, but does provide objective evidence that something is wrong. Underperformance is usually noticed too late and serial measurements of blood concentrations of haemoglobin and creatine kinase, and of packed cell volume do not help. Good diet, full hydration, and rest between training sessions will help athletes tolerate hard training. Those with a full-time job and other commitments will not recover as quickly as those who can relax after training. There are no objective tests to predict which athletes are going to break down during a period of hard training,

---

Signs of over-reaching (normal if athletes recover quickly)
- High serum creatine kinase concentration
- Low ratio of serum testosterone to cortisol concentrations
- Falls in muscle glycogen concentration
- Raised resting heart rate
- Mood deterioration

Exclusion of other causes of chronic fatigue
- History—inquire about infection, wheeze, eating disorders, chest pain, and shortness of breath on exercise
- Examination—to exclude a medical cause
- Investigation—depends on clinical possibilities. May include lung function and laboratory tests

---

Overtraining may cause immunosuppression by
- Raised serum cortisol concentrations
- Low serum glutamine concentrations
- Low salivary IgA concentrations
- Reduced T Helper: suppressor cells ratios

Laboratory tests rarely help in the diagnosis of chronic fatigue

---

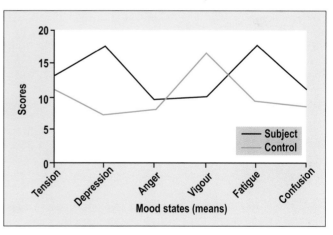

Figure 7.5 Profile of mood state (POMS) graph showing normal iceberg profile and abnormal inverted iceberg profile in overtrained athletes

---

Early detection of overtraining syndrome is difficult
- Monitor
  - performance
  - mood state
  - resting heart rate

so adequate time has to be allowed for all of them to recover. Periodisation of training should permit this, with particular care at times of intensive interval training and hard monotonous training.

Management

The treatment of any chronic fatigue syndrome requires a holistic approach and athletes are no exception. Rest and regeneration strategies are central to recovery. Five weeks of rest appreciably improve both performance and mood state, and there is growing evidence that a very low level of exercise will speed recovery.

Thus athletes must exercise aerobically (but not so hard that they cannot talk) for a few minutes each day and slowly build this up over many weeks. The level will depend on the clinical picture and rate of improvement, and recovery generally takes 6–12 weeks. Many make the mistake of trying to do a normal training session, suffering from severe fatigue for several days before partially recovering, and then do it again. Cross training (playing another sport) may be the only way of avoiding the tendency to increase the intensity too fast. Once athletes can tolerate 20 minutes of light exercise each day, then it is useful to introduce short sprints of less than 10 seconds with at least 3 minutes recovery between each sprint, two to three times per week.

Regeneration strategies are widely used in the old Eastern Bloc countries, although there are no controlled trials of treatment. They consist of rest and relaxation with counselling and psychotherapy. Massage and hydrotherapy are used and nutrition is looked at in detail. Large quantities of vitamins and supplements are given, although there is no evidence of their effectiveness. Any stresses outside sport are reduced as far as possible.

There is one report of the use of anabolic steroids (which are banned in athletes) in an attempt to speed recovery, but drugs are not generally of value unless depression is a major factor.

Athletes are often surprised at the performance they can produce after 12 weeks of extremely light exercise, and it is then that care must be taken not to increase training too fast. They need to train hard to go faster, but they must rest and recover completely at least once a week to benefit from all their hard work.

Management of the overtraining syndrome

- Relaxation strategies and rest, with regular, very light, exercise
- Communication with the coach
- Strong reassurance that the prognosis is good
- Very short sprints with long rests as condition improves

Overtrained athletes v patients with chronic fatigue

- Their primary presenting complaint is of under-performance, which is an objective measure of their condition
- They present earlier, are less severely affected and recover more quickly
- The main stresses in their lives are exercise and competition, which can be controlled
- The main problem in rehabilitation is in holding them back, rather than having to encourage appropriate exercise

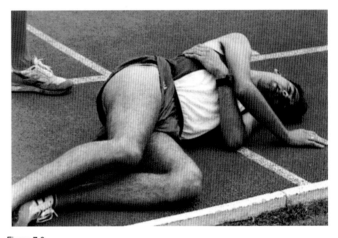

Figure 7.6

8 Sudden death

W S Hillis, P D McIntyre, J MacLean, J F Goodwin, W J McKenna

Most sudden deaths in sport are caused by cardiovascular conditions. The cardiovascular benefits of exercise are well established and epidemiology studies suggest that long-term exercise programmes may reduce the risk of sudden death. Increasing leisure time and facilities promote sports participation at all ages. A few people are at risk of serious arrhythmia or sudden death with exercise. The cause of death varies with the age of the participants; congenital structural abnormalities occur in younger age groups and coronary artery disease in older age (>35 years). Identifying such abnormalities increases the possibilities of prevention. Guidelines have been drawn up by Cardiovascular Task Forces to provide guidance concerning the advisability of exercise in patients with structural or functional abnormalities (Task Forces, 1994).

Sudden death in sport is uncommon, with an incidence of 2 cases per 100 000 subject years. Five in 100 000 athletes have a condition that might predispose them to serious cardiac problems, and of those at risk 10% (1 in 2 000 000) may die suddenly or unexpectedly (Epstein and Maron, 1986; McCaffrey et al, 1991). Considerable controversy exists about the cost effectiveness of screening all young people by examination before participation. Most criticism has been levelled at systems routinely advocating echocardiographic screening of the apparently symptomless population. Alternative views suggest targeting people with a family history of sudden death or premature coronary artery disease and educating all sports participants to seek medical advice about even minor warning symptoms.

Symptoms and signs on clinical examination suggest some cardiac causes of sudden death. The importance of others may be established only by detailed cardiological investigations. These include: electrocardiography, chest radiography, echocardiography, Doppler cardiography and, rarely, cardiac catheterisation. Exercise testing is of major value and 24–48 hour tape electrocardiographic recordings (Holter monitoring) may be required. Potentially serious symptoms, such as syncope, pre-syncope, palpitation, chest pain, and undue dyspnoea are indications that a detailed clinical history should be taken, a detailed examination should be made and, if appropriate, the patient should be referred for cardiological investigation. A family history of cardiac abnormality suggests a hereditary basis.

Coronary artery disease is the most common condition leading to sudden death during exercise, **especially** in those over 35 years of age. Death in younger athletes is rare, but may be due to hypertrophic cardiomyopathy, congenital abnormalities of the coronary artery tree, right ventricular dysplasia, valvular heart disease, such as aortic stenosis, and Marfan syndrome.

Consensus discussions have suggested classification into high and low intensity sports, with further differentiation into those with major dynamic and static components (Mitchell et al, 1994). Most cardiovascular risk occurs in those sports with extreme exertion and high dynamic demands, such as marathon running, cross-country running, skiing, basketball, football, hockey, and

> **Cardiac causes of sudden death in sport**
> - Coronary artery disease
> - Hypertrophic cardiomyopathy
> - Idiopathic concentric left ventricular hypertrophy
> - Congenital anomalies of coronary arteries
> - Aortic rupture
> - Right ventricular dysplasia
> - Myocarditis
> - Valvular disease
> - Arrhythmias and conduction defects
> - Congenital heart disease, operated or unoperated
> (Epstein and Maron, 1986)

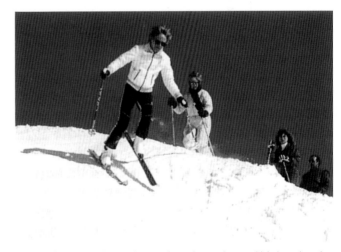

Figure 8.1 Skiing is a high intensity sport that makes moderate or high dynamic and static demands

track sports. Individuals identified as at risk should be directed to sports with low dynamic and static demands.

Contact and non-contact sports must be distinguished and activities that may place a person in jeopardy if syncope occurs should be identified. Patients with a prosthetic cardiac valve should not participate in contact sports because of potential valve dehiscence during forceful chest contact and the risks of trauma in the presence of anticoagulant drugs (Medical Conditions, 1994).

Coronary artery disease

Coronary artery disease is the major cause of sudden death in older athletes (i.e., those aged over 35 years). The risks are increasing as more middle-aged and older people participate in organised, competitive sport that requires vigorous physical exertion. During exercise, metabolic and physical changes occur that lead to an increased risk. Even in conditioned older people, sudden death may be precipitated by occult coronary atheroma. Most deaths occur in competitive long distance running and other vigorous sports, such as rugby, soccer, and squash.

History and risk factors
Previous symptoms that may suggest coronary atherosclerosis have often been recognised and risk factors are frequently present. These include smoking, a family history of myocardial infarction at under 55 years, hypertension and hyper-cholesterolaemia. The victims are often perceived as being very fit and may have competitive personalities.

Pathology
In pathological studies, obstructive atheromatous coronary artery lesions are usually found, often associated with thrombus. The myocardium may show previous unrecognised healed infarcts.

Prevention
Extreme forms of conditioning, including marathon running, do not prevent severe atherosclerosis or sudden death. Education should be emphasised to increase awareness of warning symptoms, such as chest pain, palpitation, or syncope. Severe exercise should be undertaken cautiously in patients over 40 years old, particularly those with risk factors.

Diagnosis
The use of electrocardiograph stress testing to detect those at risk may have significant limitations. In addition, the incidence of false positives may be as high as 25% in sportsmen. People should be assessed in terms of their functional capacity and risk factors.

Degree of risk
Subjects with known coronary artery disease can be classified as being at low, moderate, or high risk by assessing left ventricular function, screening for evidence of reversible ischaemia and comparing with the normal exercise capacity for age. Exercise testing may also detect ventricular arrhythmias or a reduced blood pressure response. High risk patients are those with decreased left ventricular systolic function at rest. Moderate risk patients are those with reduced exercise capacity for age, evidence of reversible ischaemia, ventricular tachycardia, or reduced systolic blood pressure. Low risk subjects with normal left ventricular function or without reversible ischaemia can participate in low intensity competitive sports, but those with moderate or high risk should be excluded. In patients who have

Classification of sports according to intensity and demands

A High intensity

1 Moderate or high dynamic and static demands

American football	Fencing	Running (sprinting)
Boxing	Ice hockey	Speed skating
Cross country skiing	Rowing	Water polo
Downhill skiing	Rugby	Wrestling

2 Moderate to high dynamic, low static demands

Badminton	Orienteering	Squash
Baseball	Race walking	Swimming
Basketball	Racket ball	Table tennis
Field hockey	Running (distance)	Tennis
Lacrosse	Soccer	Volleyball

3 Low dynamic, moderate to high static demands

Archery	Field events (jumping and throwing)	Motor cycling
Auto racing		Sailing
Diving		Ski jumping
Equestrian events	Gymnastics	Water skiing
	Karate or judo	Weight lifting

B Low intensity, low dynamic and static demands

Bowling	Curling	Shooting
Cricket	Golf	

(Mitchell *et al*, 1994)

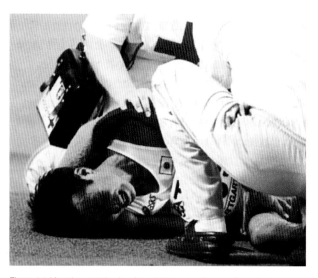

Figure 8.2 Marathon running involves extreme exertion, predisposing to musculoskeletal fatigue and potential cardiovascular collapse

Classification of sports according to danger of body collision

Contact sport	Non-contact sport	
American football	Auto racing	Ski jumping
Boxing	Bicycling	Water polo
Ice hockey	Diving	Water skiing
Karate or judo	Downhill skiing	Weight lifting
Lacrosse	Equestrian events	(increased risk if
Rugby	Gymnastics	syncope occurs)
Soccer	Motor cycling	
Wrestling	Polo	

Modified from *Pediatrics*, 1994

had coronary artery bypass grafting or angioplasty, serial assessment after the procedure should be undertaken.

Hypertrophic cardiomyopathy

Hypertrophic cardiomyopathy is the leading cause of sudden death in young athletes. The incidence of the echocardiographic features of this condition has been found in 1 in 500 of young adults (Maron et al, 1995).

Anatomical abnormalities

A hypertrophied, non-dilated left ventricle exists, but there is no history of predisposing diseases. The left ventricular chamber size is reduced and the muscular hypertrophy impairs diastolic filling. Left ventricular outflow tract obstruction may be secondary to hypertrophy of the subaortic septum, or to systolic anterior motion of the mitral valve. There are predispositions to supraventricular and ventricular arrhythmias; ventricular tachycardia may lead to ventricular fibrillation.

Cause

Hypertrophic cardiomyopathy is inherited as an autosomal dominant condition that has a high degree of penetrance. When it is identified in an individual, screening of all first degree relatives should be considered.

Symptoms

Patients may present with chest pain, palpitation, syncope or breathlessness, or may be asymptomatic. Abnormal cardiac findings may consist of a jerky or bisferiens pulse or an increased or double left ventricular apical impulse with a palpable fourth heart sound and a systolic murmur at the lower left sternal border that is decreased by squatting and increased by standing. The electrocardiogram is usually abnormal, although the findings may be non-specific. Cardiomegaly may be present on chest radiography, but the diagnosis is made on echocardiography, which shows a small cavity and hypertrophy of the left ventricle, limited compliance, and limited diastolic filling.

Future exercise

The presence of cardiomyopathy should restrict people from engaging in strenuous dynamic exercise sports, but those at low risk may follow a moderate exercise programme.

Differentiation from "athletic heart"

Left ventricular hypertrophy is common as a normal response to training, but the ventricular wall is rarely more than 12 mm thick. A thickness of more than 16 mm is strongly suggestive of hypertrophic cardiomyopathy.

Other causes

Congenital coronary artery abnormalities

Patients may present with symptoms of anginal pain, syncope with exertion, or even sudden death. This may be associated with anomalous origin of the left coronary artery, which is constricted by the aorta during exercise. Investigations should include a 12-lead electrocardiogram, a two dimensional echocardiogram to assess the position of origin of the left main coronary artery, and an exercise stress test.

Prognostic factors for sudden death caused by hypertrophic cardiomyopathy

- Family history of sudden death
- Documented ventricular tachycardia
- Young age at onset of symptoms

(Fanapazir et al, 1992)

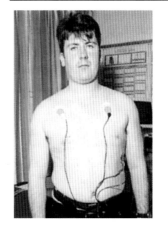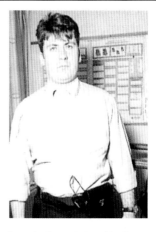

Figure 8.3 During 24–48 hour tape electrocardiography; the contacts and leads are covered by clothing and the recorder fixed to the belt

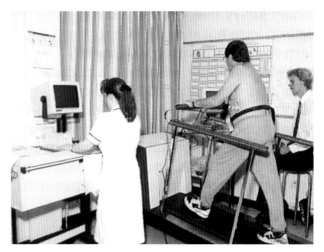

Figure 8.4 Exercise testing is useful to diagnose many cardiac disorders

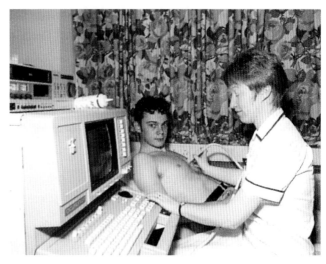

Figure 8.5 Echocardiography is the diagnostic test for hypertrophic cardiomyopathy

Marfan syndrome

The body habitus of affected individuals may help participation in sport, such as basketball and volleyball. Cardiovascular involvement gives mitral valve prolapse in almost all patients. The risk of aortic involvement is variable, but requires serial review. If the syndrome is suspected on clinical appearance and by the presence of a family history the patient should be referred for regular echocardiography. Beta blockers should be prescribed to retard the rate of aortic root dilatation and given to all patients, including those with dilated aortic roots and those who have had aortic surgery.

Right ventricular dysplasia (Corrado, 1998)

Right ventricular cardiomyopathy or dysplasia has been reported as a cause of sudden death during sport and may have a regional geographical distribution in the north of Italy. It is associated with fibrous, fatty replacement of the right ventricular myocardium, which is grossly dilated.

Myocarditis

Occasional sports-specific reports have identified unusual conditions in local populations, and sudden death associated with myocarditis was noted among young Swedish orienteers (Wesslen et al, 1996). These observations led to a six month intermission in training and competition, with strict exclusion of individuals participating who had evidence of ongoing infection.

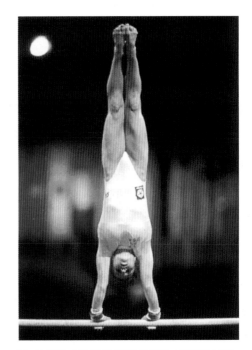

Figure 8.6 Gymnastics is a high intensity sport that makes low dynamic and moderate to high static demands

Valvular disease

Aortic stenosis

Symptoms of left ventricular failure, syncope, or anginal pain from aortic stenosis occur late. In those with a symptomatic, mild to moderate stenosis, participation may occur in low intensity sports (Class B) or, alternatively, moderate static or dynamic demands (Class A3).

Mitral valve prolapse

Mitral valve prolapse may occur in up to 6% of the normal population. In the absence of symptoms and signs, or associated lesions, and with a negative family history, full sporting participation should be allowed. In the presence of palpitations, dizziness, or near syncope, both Holter monitoring and stress testing are invaluable for assessment of the mechanism of the symptoms. Associated problems that might exclude sporting activity include an associated prolonged QT syndrome, or a family history of sudden death associated with a mitral valve prolapse (Jeresaty, 1986).

Valve replacement

In patients who have had valvuloplasty or annuloplasty, contact sports should be avoided. Athletes with a prosthetic valve and normal cardiac function may engage in low intensity sports.

Arrhythmias

Arrhythmias in young people may be associated with structural cardiac abnormalities, operated or unoperated, or have an inherent predisposition. Routine electrocardiographic screening will identify those with Wolff-Parkinson-White syndrome and those with the long QT syndrome (Garson et al, 1993).

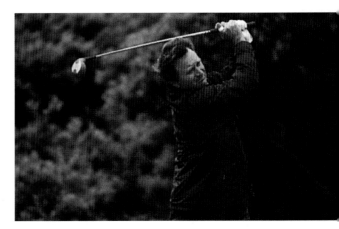

Figure 8.7 Golf is a low intensity sport with little danger of body collision

Congenital heart disease

It is most important that advice regarding the advisability of exercise in individuals with adult congenital heart disease be formulated. Individuals with previous operations, particularly right ventriculotomy, may be predisposed to significant arrhythmias. Individual assessment must be undertaken.

Screening issues

Several issues regarding screening remain controversial. The first circumstantial evidence that a screening programme can impact on mortality during sport has been produced following 20 years of active screening in Italy (Corrado *et al*, 1998). This programme, utilising a health questionnaire, physical examination and ECG, has identified those with hypertrophic cardiomyopathy and excluded them from competitive sport. Comparative data with other countries suggest that this protective policy has reduced mortality in this patient group. The challenge remains for each health care system to make available appropriate facilities for those participants who would wish to volunteer for cardiac screening.

> **Issues requiring further study**
> - Identifying causes of sudden death during physical exercise
> - The appropriateness, cost, and practicality of cardiovascular screening of presumably healthy children and adolescents before they participate in sport, and of other people before they continue or return to sport
> - Counselling patients with known cardiac abnormalities about their levels of activity and about the risk and safety of specific sporting events
> - Establishing guidelines for disqualification from competition

References

Anon (1994) Medical conditions affecting sporting participation. *Pediatrics* **94**(5): 757–60

Corrado D, Basso C, Sciavon M, Thiene G (1998) Screening for hypertrophic cardiomyopathy in young athletes. *N Engl J Med* **339**: 365–9

Epstein SE, Maron BJ (1986) Sudden death and the competitive athlete: perspectives on pre-participating screening studies. *J Am Coll Cardiol* **7**: 220–30

Fanapazir L, Chang AC, Epstein SE, McAreavy D (1992) Prognostic determinants in hypertrophic cardiomyopathy. *Circulation* **86**: 730–40

Garson A, MacDonald D, Fournier A, *et al* (1993) The long QT syndrome in children. *Circulation* **87**: 1866–72

Jevesaty RM (1986) Mitral valve prolapse: definitions and implications in athletes. *J Am Coll Cardiol* **7**(1): 231–6

Maron BJ, Gardin JM, Flack JM, Gidding SS, Kurosaki TT, Bild DE (1995) Prevalence of hypertrophic cardiomyopathy in a general population of young adults. *Circulation* **92**: 785–9

McCaffrey FM, Braden DS, Strong WB (1991) Sudden cardiac death in young athletes. *Am J Dis Child* **145**: 177–83

Mitchell JH, Haskell WC, Raven PB (1994) Classification of sports. *J Am Coll Cardiol* **24**(4): 864–6

Task Forces (1994) 1. Congenital Heart Disease, 2. Acquired Valvular Heart Disease, 3. Hypertrophic Cardiomyopathy, 4. Hypertension, 5. Coronary Artery Disease. *J Am Coll Cardiol* **24**(4): 845–99

Wesslen L, Pahlson C, Lindquist O, *et al* (1996) An increase in sudden unexpected cardiac deaths among young Swedish orienteers during 1979–1992. *Eur Heart J* **17**: 902–10

9 Setting up an exercise laboratory in a general hospital

Richard Godfrey

Introduction

Regular exercise is increasingly recognised by the medical profession as being effective in preventing disease and enhancing quality of life. The role of exercise in health and fitness is best assessed with regular monitoring of a number of indices of physiological function, one important example being "physical work capacity". The asessment can be made using one of a variety of laboratory-based exercise testing modalities. This chapter describes how to set up an exercise laboratory in the hospital environment and provides a few ideas on the appropriate use of various assessment protocols in such a setting.

Table 9.1: Wish list for equipping an exercise laboratory in a hospital setting

Equipment	Necessary	Desirable
Treadmill	✔	
Bicycle ergometer	✔	
On-line gas analysis system	✔	
12-lead ECG	✔	
3-lead ECG		✔
Enzymatic lactate analyser		✔
On-line spirometer	✔	
Hand grip dynamometer		✔
Isokinetic loading dynamometer		✔
Fluid-filled goniometer		✔
Skinfold calipers	✔	
Weighing scales	✔	
Stadiometer	✔	
Water cooler	✔	
Defibrillator	✔	
Air conditioning unit + ventilation	✔	

How much space is needed ?

As the title of the latest American College of Sports Medicine Position Stand suggests, the major investment should be made in testing cardiorespiratory and muscular fitness and flexibility. A plan of the main laboratory at the British Olympic Medical Centre (BOMC) is shown in *Figure 9.1*, while *Figure 9.2* shows a suggested layout ideal for a general hospital exercise laboratory using less than half that space. Much of the equipment in the BOMC is used to test elite athletes and may not be suitable if space is at a

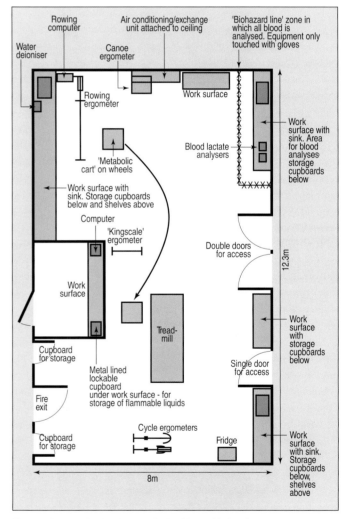

Figure 9.1 Layout of main laboratory, British Olympic Medical Centre

premium. A minimum ceiling height of 3 m is essential to allow full elevation of most treadmills with a tall individual exercising.

Extensive work surface, a sink, separate cupboard space for consumables and cleaning materials, and a further 'stand-alone' metal-lined cupboard for inflammable liquids, such as alcohol, are all needed. The laboratory should be fully air-conditioned and ventilated in order to maintain ideal ambient conditions.

A mobile 'on-line' cardiopulmonary gas exchange system or 'metabolic cart' is most practical for measuring the subject's oxygen consumption and carbon dioxide output during exercise. A 12-lead ECG monitor is essential but a 3-lead ECG monitor is also recommended. A number of choices are available for strength testing and this will be discussed more fully later. A couch is useful for subject preparation. Also needed are weighing scales, height measure and a flow–volume loop system to measure both static and dynamic lung function. A water cooler or other source of drinking water is essential. At the BOMC food and drink in the laboratory is forbidden, but there is one exception. Athletes being tested can drink fluids at the discretion of staff present. An automatic defibrillator is essential. Staff conducting exercise tests must be holders of a current certificate in basic life support from the Resuscitation Council (UK).

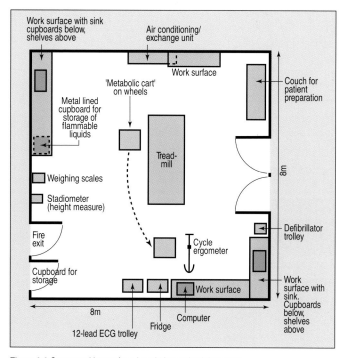

Figure 9.2 Suggested layout for a hospital exercise laboratory

Ergometry

Ideally, both a treadmill and stationary cycle ergometer are required. For the average individual, the treadmill is a better test ergometer as assessment of aerobic power associated with running and walking exercise is most consistent with everyday activity. However, patients with physical problems that preclude weight-bearing should be exercised on a cycle ergometer. Many ergometers can be controlled by the metabolic cart and, in a hospital setting, this is the recommended set-up. A mechanically braked bike would require the tester to change the load periodically. This would require calculation beforehand of the loads required at each stage and changing the load during testing can prove awkward. An electrically braked bike controlled by the metabolic cart will automatically increase the resistance according to the preset protocol. This also means it is far easier for one individual to administer the test without help.

Measurement of cardiopulmonary gas exchange (CPX)

The method most commonly used for measuring aerobic power is referred to as 'indirect calorimetry' and values are obtained by comparing the gas composition of expired air with that of ambient air. The rate of oxygen consumed can be calculated from the difference between these two if the volume of air breathed each minute is accurately measured, usually using a turbine or pneumotachograph.

Gas analysis is performed using a CO_2 analyser (usually infra-red), which samples expired air and determines CO_2 content, and an O_2 analyser (usually paramagnetic, zirconium oxide, or oxygen electrode [based on the Clark principle]).

A central processing unit (CPU) integrates the information and gives 'real-time' graphical display of the 'breath-by-breath' expired gas volumes and flow rates. In addition, a print-out of a range of ventilatory data at user-specified time points can be obtained and graphs plotted. The gas analysers, flow measurement equipment and CPU are housed together and known generically as a cardiopulmonary gas exchange system, metabolic measurement system or 'metabolic cart' (*Figure 9.3*).

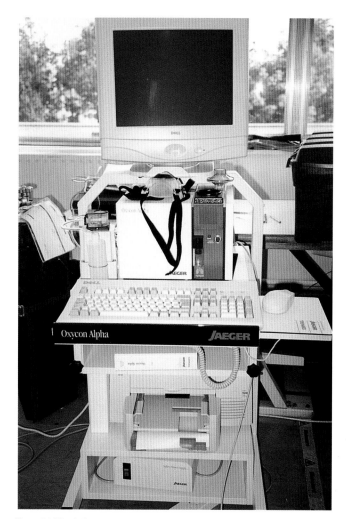

Figure 9.3 Metabolic cart

Most metabolic carts can be purchased with a 12-lead ECG machine and this is a highly recommended option for use in a clinical setting. Integration of 12-lead ECG and oxygen consumption measurement will allow impairment of function to be characterised. The percentage of functional aerobic impairment can be calculated from the following equation:

$$\%FAI = \frac{predicted\ VO_2\max - observed\ VO_2\max}{predicted\ VO_2\max} \times 100$$

Strength assessment

Hand-grip dynamometer

An estimate of whole body strength can be made in sedentary to moderately active people using the hand-grip dynamometer (*Figure 9.4*). The equipment allows repeatable measurements and a large amount of normal data already exists with which to make comparisons. However, for elite athletes or individuals who weight train, grip strength is less useful as an index of whole body strength.

Isokinetic loading dynamometer *(Figure 9.5)*

This type of equipment is very expensive and is probably best housed within a physiotherapy department. The machine consists of chair with a a lever arm to which the limb or body part to be assessed is strapped. The maximum speed that the lever arm can be moved is fixed at a set speed. The patient is asked to attempt three maximal effort extensions and flexions of the limb. The speed that the lever arm can be moved at can be set, the muscles involved in the movement tested and then a new speed can be selected. Providing the patient performs a maximal effort, the strength of the active muscle groups can be measured at the set speed. Generally, four different speeds are selected and so the muscle groups can be assessed through a range of functional speeds. The advantage is that muscle strength imbalances can be identified and subsequently corrected. In addition, the equipment can be used to measure and facilitate rehabilitation from injury.

Disadvantages of this equipment include purchase cost, its large size, and lack of portability. Additionally, this equipment is not specific enough to assess changes in strength and power that relate to sports performance. The equipment does not allow accelerations and decelerations that form the basis of most sports movements. However, this control of movement speed makes it a useful rehabilitation tool as accelerations and decelerations often exacerbate existing injuries.

Flexibility assessment

Ideally, this is carried out by a physiotherapist using a fluid-filled goniometer. Range of movement can be assessed around a number of different joints. Daily exercises can be prescribed to improve range of movement if flexibility is poor.

Body composition assessment

A measurement of height and of body mass is required. Height is measured using a stadiometer and body mass using a reliable beam balance or electronic weighing machine. If an accurate and precise measure of body fat is required, the method that is fast gaining acceptance as the 'Gold Standard' is DEXA (Dual Emission X-ray Absorbitometry). This allows differentiation of

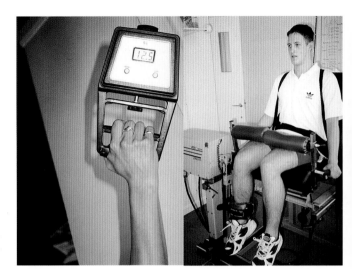

Figure 9.4 Hand-grip dynamometer

Figure 9.5 Isokinetic loading dynamometer

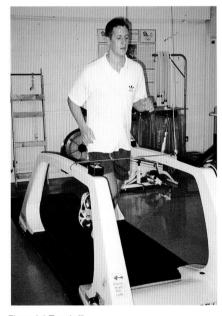

Figure 9.6 Treadmill

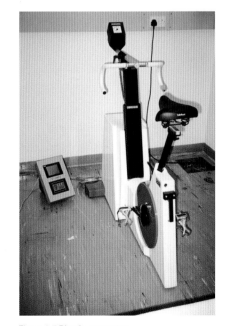

Figure 9.7 Bicycle ergometer

body mass into three major components; muscle, fat, and bone. In addition, it has the advantage of allowing regional fat deposition to be seen. The disadvantage of this method is cost and that it requires trained, experienced personnel to operate the equipment and interpret the results.

The most commonly applied, and arguably the best, practical method of determining body composition is the use of skinfold calipers. There are several assumptions inherent in this method. However, if the same individual makes the measurements in a standardised way on each occasion then the trend in changes in body composition can be followed over time. Hence this method can achieve a good degree of precision, but does sacrifice accuracy. In the UK generally, the four skinfold site method of Durnin and Womersley (1974) is used.

Protocols to determine aerobic power

Many individuals who are inexperienced in conducting exercise tests worry about the risks of testing sedentary or unfit subjects to maximal exercise. In fact, the risks of fatality are very small at around 1 in 20,000 subjects tested (ACSM, 1995).

Treadmill

The Bruce protocol is one of the most commonly chosen to test clinical subjects and involves exercising to volitional exhaustion. The major advantages of this test are the large amount of normal data that have accumulated and the rigorous validation it has undergone over the years.

Bicycle ergometer (*Figure 9.7*)

A maximal test can be used or, if there is genuine and justifiable concern about testing an individual to maximal heart rate, a predictive test can be applied.

An example of a predictive test is the PWC170 bicycle ergometer test that involves exercising at three submaximal workloads in a continuous manner. Each at a progressively higher intensity. The final effort should elicit a heart-rate of around 170 beats/min[-1]. The test relies upon the fact that there is a linear relationship between heart rate (HR) and oxygen consumption in submaximal exercise. At higher intensities HR begins to plateau as it approaches its maximum. Submaximal HR and oxygen consumption is measured and plotted on a graph. Using the Karvonen formula (220-age) to predict maximal achievable HR the graph of HR vs VO_2 can be extrapolated to cross a line drawn perpendicular to the predicted maximal heart rate on the y axis. A line is then drawn down to the x axis from the intersection between the extrapolated graph and the line corresponding to the predicted maximal heart rate to obtain a prediction for VO_2max (*Figure 9.8*).

When is a max a "true" max ?

To be termed maximal oxygen uptake (VO_2max) the individual must achieve volitional exhaustion between 9–15 minutes and achieve most of the criteria listed. If a VO_2 associated with a maximal effort has a duration of less than 8 minutes or greater than 12 minutes it is generally termed 'VO_2 peak'.

Bruce Protocol. Patient exercises until volitional exhaustion and VO2max is estimated from equation:
VO2max = [6.7-2.82(sex; m=1, f=2) + 0.056 x (Time in seconds)

Stage	Speed (km/h)	Gradient (%)	Time (minutes)
I	2.7	10	0–3
II	4.0	12	3–6
III	5.4	14	6–9
IV	6.7	16	9–12
V	8.0	18	12–15
VI	8.8	20	15–18
VII	9.6	22	18–21

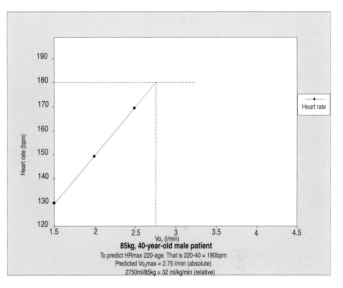

85kg, 40-year-old male patient
To predict HRmax 220-age. That is 220-40 = 180bpm
Predicted Vo₂max = 2.75 l/min (absolute)
2750ml/85kg = 32 ml/kg/min (relative)

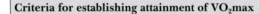

Figure 9.8 PWC₁₇₀ Bicycle ergonometer test

Criteria for establishing attainment of VO₂max

- HR within 5–10 beats of predicted maximum
- a plateau on the O₂ consumption curve (i.e. no more than 2 ml/kg/min difference over the last three points)
- an RER greater than 1.15
- a plasma lactate of greater than 8 mM

Lactate profiling

There is a growing body of research evidence suggesting that exercise at, or just above, the lactate threshold is one of the most effective training areas for many circumstances. Exercise just above threshold has been shown to be effective in improving insulin sensitivity in non-insulin dependent diabetic patients, in weight loss, in improving mood state and sense of well-being, in reducing the magnitude of the decline in physical work capacity normally associated with ageing and in improving performance in top class athletes.

In order to establish the lactate threshold, a discontinuous incremental, or "step" test is applied. The subject is asked to warm up and is then exercise, for example,d on the treadmill with heart rate and oxygen consumption being measured on-line throughout the whole test. The test begins at a low intensity for four minutes. A 30 second gap allows a small arterialised blood sample to be taken from the earlobe or fingertip. The next four minutes requires exercise at 1km/h faster and then again a capillary blood sample is taken. This process of four minutes of exercise, each at increasing intensity with a 30 second gap after each is continued until the subject is unable to complete four minutes at a given treadmill velocity. The whole blood samples can be analysed using an enzymatic analyser and a graph plotted of lactate vs treadmill velocity. The inflexion point on the resulting curve is the lactate threshold (*Figure 9.9*), and the subject can be given a heart rate range at which to exercise corresponding to this point. Any exercise programme will, therefore, consist of training that includes a balance of low intensity exercise of 30–60 minutes duration and 'threshold' exercise of 20–40 minutes duration. Improvements can be charted if the subject is retested two to three months later by a 'rightward shift' in the lactate curve (*Figure 9.10*) That is a lower blood lactate at the same submaximal exercise intensity.

Summary

Determine

- The range of tests that are to be catered for
- What equipment is to be used
- How much room equipment will take up in lab during both use and storage.

Ensure

- You plan the lab layout. Draw the floor-plan, including a safe working area around each item of equipment
- There is adequate cupboard space
- There is a separate, metal lined cupboard for flammable liquids
- There is a sink and work surface provided
- Adequate ventilation and air conditioning
- There is a defibrillator in the lab and that all staff are competent in its use.

References

American College of Sports Medicine (1998) *ACSM Resource Manual for Guidelines for Exercise Testing and Prescription*, 3rd edn. Williams and Wilkins, Philadelphia

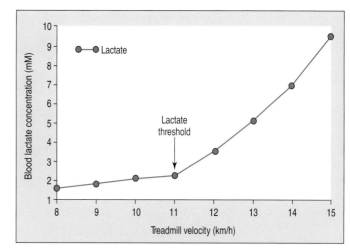

Figure 9.9 Graph of blood lactate concentration against treadmill velocity showing lactate threshold

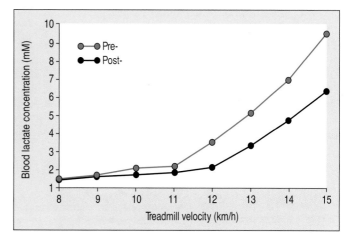

Figure 9.10 Graph showing rightward shift in the lactate curve after 8–12 weeks of threshold training

American College of Sports Medicine (1998) Position Stand The Recommended Quantity and Quality of Exercise for Developing and Maintaining Cardiorespiratory and Muscular Fitness, and Flexibility in Healthy Adults. *Med Sci Sports Exerc* **30**(6): 975–91

American College of Sports Medicine (1995) *ACSM Guidelines for Exercise Testing and Prescription*, 5th edition. Williams and Wilkins, Philadelphia

Durnin JV, Womersley J (1974) Body fat assessed from total body density and its estimation from skinfold thickness measurements on 481 men and women aged 16 to 72 years. *Br J Nutr* **32**: 77–97.

Further reading

Bird S, Davison R, eds (1997) *BASES Physiological Testing Guidelines*, 3rd edn. British Association of Sport and Exercise Sciences, Leeds

Harries M, Williams C, Stanish WD, Micheli LJ, eds (1998) *Oxford Textbook of Sports Medicine*, 2nd edn. Oxford University Press, Oxford

10 Drugs in sport

Andrea Daly

Citius, Altius, Fortius—swiftest, highest, strongest translates the Olympic motto. To be the best is surely the ambition of every sportsperson; in some cases, however, it is at a cost to themselves and to the reputation of their sport.

The enhancement of performance in sport by the use of chemical agents is termed doping. Doping is against the rules and ethics of both sport and medical science and is deemed cheating. Therefore, in the UK, doping control is undertaken by the UK Sports Council to ensure fair competition and protect the health of athletes. Drug testing is used to deter athletes from using ergogenic substances or methods, to detect doping offences, and to demonstrate that the majority of athletes are drug-free.

Most governing bodies in sport abide by the rules set down by the International Olympic Committee Medical Code. This can be subdivided into three sections.

Prohibited classes of substances

Unless specifically indicated, all substances belonging to the banned classes (including veterinary products) may not be used even if they are not listed as examples. Hence the term 'related substances' is used to describe drugs that are related by their pharmacological actions and/or chemical structure.

Prohibited methods

These include:

- blood doping
- pharmacological, chemical, and physical manipulation—for example, the use of probenecid as a masking agent.

Classes of drugs subject to certain restrictions

Although not totally prohibited, the use of drugs in this category may lead to action being taken upon a positive test in certain sports.

The anti-anxiety effect of β-blockers could enhance performance in certain sports, such as the bobsleigh, ski jumping, and shooting events (including the modern pentathlon) and for this reason they are banned. There are a wide range of effective alternatives to β-blockers available in order to control hypertension, cardiac arrhythmias, angina, and migraine.

In contrast, it is the route of administration that determines whether or not corticosteroids are prohibited. Their use is banned, except for topical use (anal, aural, dermatological, nasal, and opthalmological), but not rectal, inhalational therapy (asthma, allergic rhinitis) and local or intra-articular injections.

International Olympic Committee Medical Code

Prohibited classes of substances and prohibited methods (January 1998)

I   **Prohibited classes of substances**
- A   Stimulants
- B   Narcotics
- C   Anabolic agents
- D   Diuretics
- E   Peptide and glycoprotein hormones and analogues

II   **Prohibited methods**
- A   Blood doping
- B   Pharmacological, chemical, and physical manipulation

III   **Classes of drugs subject to certain restrictions**
- A   Alcohol
- B   Marijuana
- C   Local anaesthetics
- D   Corticosteroids
- E β-Blockers

Doctors need to provide prior written notice if they wish to administer corticosteroids by inhalation or by local or intra-articular injection to a competitor. It is believed these restrictions do not interfere with the normal medical, mainly anti-inflammatory, uses of these compounds.

With the exception of cocaine, all local anaesthetics are allowed when medically justified. However, only local or intra-articular injections may be administered. Cocaine is banned under all circumstances.

Testing

Due to the abuse of drugs to enhance training effects and subsequent performance in competition, testing in some sports has been extended to take place at any time. During training, anabolic agents, peptide hormones, and manipulation techniques are most likely to be abused, while drugs to improve 'on-the-day' performance, such as stimulants, β-blockers, and diuretics, are more likely during competition.

Prohibited drug classes

Stimulants

The treatment of asthma and upper respiratory ailments with β_2-adrenoceptor agents are well established, however, their use in sport is controlled and restricted. The I.O.C. permits the use of salbutamol, terbutaline and, more recently, salmeterol by inhaler only. All other dosage preparations of β_2-adrenoceptors are banned as stimulants. The use of sodium chromoglycate, theophylline, choline theophyllinate and aminophylline is unrestricted. It should also be remembered that many over-the-counter preparations contain the stimulant, caffeine. Solpadeine®, a combined analgesic, contains 30 mg of caffeine in each tablet/capsule and Feminax®, which may be purchased by female athletes for the relief of dysmenorrhoea, contains 50 mg of caffeine in each tablet. These are just a few examples to highlight the need for verification with the pharmacist by the athlete.

Narcotics

Analgesics are one of the most commonly prescribed drug classes by doctors for sportsmen and women. The use of narcotic analgesics is restricted due to their ergogenic effects of masking pain and inducing euphoria. In such instances where severe pain was apparent, their use could be warranted provided no competition was undertaken. All nonsteroidal anti-inflammatory drugs are allowed for the relief of pain. Where their use is contraindicated, codeine or a combined analgesic, such as paracetamol and dextropropoxyphene (co-proxamol), could be used. Dextromethorphan and pholcodine, active ingredients in many mixtures for dry cough, and diphenoxylate, used in the treatment of diarrhoea, are all allowed.

Anabolic agents

This class includes both anabolic–androgenic steroids and β_2 agonists; the latter when administered systemically are thought to have powerful anabolic properties. Inadvertent use of anabolic–androgenic steroids is unlikely due to their limited therapeutic indications. Stanozolol can be used for pruritis associated with obstructive jaundice in palliative care. Androgens, such as testosterone, are occasionally used in metastatic breast cancer and in replacement therapy in male hypogonadism. These restricted clinical uses highlight the unlikelihood of anabolic

---

Stimulants

Includes the following examples:

Amineptine	Fencamfamine
Amiphenazole	Mesocarb
Amphetamines	Pentylentetrazol
Bromantan	Pipradol
Caffeine*	Salbutamol***
Carphedon	Salmeterol***
Cocaine	Terbutaline***
Ephedrines**	. . . and related substances

*For caffeine the definition of a positive result depends on the concentration of caffeine in the urine. The concentration in urine may not exceed 12 micrograms per millilitre

** For ephedrine, caffeine, and methylephedrine, the definition of a positive is 5 micrograms per millilitre of urine. For phenylpropanolamine and pseudoephedrine the definition of a positive is 10 micrograms per millilitre. If more than one of these substances is present, the quantities should be added and, if the sum exceeds 10 micrograms per millilitre, the sample should be considered positive

*** Permitted by inhaler only when their use is previously certified in writing by a respiratory or team physician to the relevant medical authority

Note: All imidazole preparations are acceptable for topical use, for example, oxymetazoline. Vasoconstrictors (for example, adrenaline) may be administered with local anaesthetic agents. Topical preparations of phenylephrine are permitted, for example, nasal, ophthalmological.

Narcotics

Includes the following examples:

Dextromoramide	Morphine
Diamorphine (heroin)	Pentazocine
Methadone	Pethidine
	. . . and related substances

Note: codeine, dextromethorphan, dextropropoxyphene, dihydrocodeine, diphenoxylate, ethylmorphine, pholcodine and propoxyphene are permitted

steroids being prescribed by doctors for healthy competitors in sport.

One drug, which for obvious reasons does not appear on the prohibited list, is insulin; unfortunately, problems of associated abuse do exist, especially in power sports. Insulin has both anabolic and anticatabolic actions and is, therefore, used as an anabolic agent, often without full awareness of the associated dangers, notably those of hypoglycaemia. The recent change of human insulin from P to POM status will, hopefully, limit this abuse for the future. Vigilance by doctors is required with regards to its supply on repeat prescriptions and by community pharmacists who may deal with requests for emergency supplies.

Diuretics

Diuretics are misused to reduce weight quickly in sports where weight restrictions apply, such as boxing, and to dilute the concentration of banned substances in urine, thereby minimising detection. In both cases health risks are involved due to the side-effects that may occur, such as electrolyte depletion and dehydration. It is for these reasons that the I.O.C. decided to include diuretics under its banned substance list. The manipulation of body weight is deemed unethical. Therefore, in sports involving weight divisions, athletes may be required to provide urine samples at the weigh in. Alternatives to diuretics, such as angiotensin-converting enzyme inhibitors or calcium channel blockers, may be used for the on-going treatment of hypertension.

Peptide and glycoprotein hormones and analogues

Choronic gonadotrophin, corticotrophin, and growth hormone are banned due to their anabolic effects, but it is unlikely that doctors would prescribe these for healthy individuals. Consequently, individuals requesting them should be viewed with caution. Erythropoietin has been demonstrated to be as effective as blood doping in the improvement of endurance capacity and maximal oxygen uptake (VO_2max). It is for these reasons that its unwarranted use constitutes doping.

Treatment of common ailments

Self-medication with over-the-counter preparations may lead to inadvertent drug misuse. Numerous cough and cold preparations contain banned ephedrine-based substances, for example, Sudafed®, Lemsip®, and Day Nurse®. Use of these products could lead to a positive test result. While all antihistamines are permitted for use, they are often found in combination with the banned sympathomimetics in such products. Preparations, such as vitamins and herbal and nutritional supplements, are perceived by the majority to be safe and innocuous. This is often not the case as some contain banned substances, such as guarana, ma huang and Chinese ephedra, which exhibit stimulant effects. Hence care must be taken and athletes should seek appropriate advice if uncertain. Cooperation between patient and practitioner is paramount and knowledge of all pharmaceutical products being used is essential.

Education

In recent years, priority has been given to raising the awareness of drugs and sport for all concerned. Governing bodies are encouraged to offer appropriate education to their members with regards to drug use, testing procedures, and the regulations involved. Increasing the awareness has, hopefully, allowed

---

Anabolic agents

I Anabolic androgenic agents

includes the following examples:

Androstenedione Metenolone
Clostebol Nandrolone
Dehydroepiandrosterone Oxandrolone
Fluoxymesterone Stanozolol
Metandienone Testosterone
. . . and related substances

II β_2-Agonists

includes the following examples:

Clenbuterol
Fenoterol
Salbutamol
Salmeterol
Terbutaline
. . . and related substances

Diuretics

includes the following examples:

Acetazolamide Hydrochlorothiazide
Bumetanide Mannitol*
Chlorthalidone Mersalyl
Ethacrynic acid Spironolactone
Furosemide Triamterene
. . . and related substances

* Prohibited by intravenous injection

Peptide and glycoprotein hormones and analogues

includes the following examples:

Chorionic gonadotrophin*
Corticotrophin*
Growth hormone*
Erythropoietin

* All respective releasing factors and their analogues are also prohibited

athletes, coaches, and doctors to make informed decisions about the taking of medicines. Education initiatives for members have included posters, advice booklets, and advice cards, The identification of education required has to be on-going and a balance between both education and testing is essential.

Conclusion

Ignorance of the rules is no defence and athletes use pharmaceutical products at their own risk. It should be remembered that not all sports adopt the I.O.C. Medical Code, so if doubt exists checks with the relevant governing body should be made. Doctors requiring assistance can refer to the information provided in the British National Formulary. The Sports Council have also made available an advice card (credit card size) that can be used as a quick reference source for athletes and doctors to carry around with them. Further detailed checks can be made with the U.K.S.C. Drug Information Line on 0171 380 8030.

The comprehensive testing and education programmes in the UK are aimed towards the prevention of doping in sport and the achievement of drug-free sport.

Summary

- Not all sports adopt the I.O.C. Medical Code, therefore, checks with governing bodies should be made when uncertainty exists
- Athletes use pharmaceutical products at their own risk
- Numerous OTC and herbal preparations contain banned substances
- Doctors can find a list of banned substances in the BNF
- Detailed checks can be made with the UKSC Information Line
- Both athletes and doctors can order the advice card from the Sports Council to use as a quick reference source
- A balance between education and testing is essential.

References

Ethics and Anti-doping Directorate (1996/7) *Annual Report*. United Kingdom Sports Council, Walkden House, London

Korkia P, Stimson GV (1997) Indications of prevalence, practice and effects of anabolic steroid use in Great Britain. *Int J Sports Med* **18**: 557–62

Schwenk TL (1997) Psychoactive drugs and athletic performane. *Phys Sportsmed* **25**(1): 32–46

Willey JW (1997) Insulin as an anabolic aid? A danger for strength athletes. *Phys Sportsmed* **25**(10): 103–4

Further reading

Bloomfield J, Fricker PA, Fritch KD (1995) *Science and Medicine in Sport*, 2nd edn. Blackwell Science, London: 590–600

Examples of permitted and prohibited substances (as issued by I.O.C. January 1998)

Asthma	Permitted	Salbutamol*, salmeterol*, terbutaline*, beclomethasone*, fluticasone*, sodium chromoglycate, theophylline (*by inhalation only)
	Prohibited	Sympathomimetics, e.g. ephedrine, isoprenaline, fenoterol, rimiterol, orciprenaline
Cold/cough	Permitted	All antibiotics, menthol and steam inhalations, products containing astemizole, terfenadine, pholcodine, guaiphenesin, dextromethorphan, paracetamol
	Prohibited	Sympathomimetics, e.g. ephedrine, pseudoephedrine, phenylpropanolamine
Diarrhoea	Permitted	Diphenoxylate, loperamide, products containing electrolytes (e.g. Dioralyte)
	Prohibited	Products containing opioids, e.g. morphine
Hayfever	Permitted	Antihistamines, nasal sprays containing xylometazoline or a corticosteroid, eye drops containing sodium chromoglycate
	Prohibited	Products containing ephedrine and pseudoephedrine
Pain	Permitted	Aspirin, codeine, dihydrocodeine, ibuprofen, paracetamol, dextropropoxyphene, all nonsteroidal anti-inflammatory drugs
	Prohibited	Products containing opioids, caffeine
Vomiting	Permitted	Domperidone, metoclopramide

11 Active in later life

Archie Young and Susie Dinan

The benefits

Introduction

Regular physical activity brings important health benefits at any age. Any potential hazards can be reduced by education and guidance of participants.

Prevention of disease

Regular physical activity helps prevent conditions important in "old age", notably, osteoporosis, non-insulin dependent diabetes mellitus, hypertension, ischaemic heart disease, probably stroke, and perhaps colonic cancer.

Prevention of disability

Not only does regular physical activity have important disease-preventing effects, its function-preserving effects are also important. Appropriate physical training improves the functional abilities of people with disabling symptoms of intermittent claudication, angina pectoris, heart failure, asthma, and chronic bronchitis. Frail, elderly patients with multiple disabilities may also derive functional benefits from graded physical training.

Even healthy elderly people lose strength (the ability to exert force) at some 1–2% per year and power (= force x speed) at some 3–4% per year. In addition, many elderly people have further problems due to the presence of chronic disease. The resulting weakness has important functional consequences for the performance of everyday activities. For example, in the English National Fitness Survey, nearly half of women and 15% of men aged 70–74 years had a power/weight ratio (for extension of the lower limb) too low to be confident of being able to mount a 30 cm step without using their hands. A similar argument applies for endurance capacity; 80% of women and 35% of men aged 70–74 years had an aerobic power/weight ratio so low that they would be unable to sustain comfortably a walk at 3 mph. Similarly, at least a third of women and 22% of men aged 70–74 years had shoulder abduction so restricted that they would be unable to wash their hair without difficulty.

Regular exercise increases strength, endurance, and flexibility. In percentage terms, the improvements seen in elderly people are similar to those in younger people. For example, in two Royal Free studies: (1) women aged 75 to 93 years increased their strength by 24–30%, equivalent to a 'rejuvenation' of strength by 15–20 years, with just 12 weeks of strength training, and (2) women aged 80 to 93 years produced a 15% mean increase in their aerobic power/weight ratio with 24 weeks of endurance training, equivalent to a "rejuvenation" of endurance of 15 years.

Prevention of immobility

For those who are severely disabled, immobility has substantial hazards. Movement, even in the absence of a training effect,

---

Physical activity helps to prevent

Disease, such as:
- Osteoporosis
- Non-insulin dependent diabetes
- Hypertension
- Ishaemic heart disease
- Stroke
- Anxiety
- Depression
- Colonic cancer?

Disability caused by:
- Intermittent claudication
- Angina pectoris
- Heart failure
- Asthma
- Chronic bronchitis
- Age related weakness

Problems, such as:
- Arthritic pain
- Poor sleep
- Falls

Immobility, which can cause:
- Faecal impaction
- Deep vein thrombosis
- Gravitational oedema

Isolation, which can cause:
- Loneliness
- Depression
- Mental lethargy

contributes to the prevention of faecal impaction, deep vein thrombosis and gravitational oedema.

Prevention of isolation

In addition to its physiological effects, recreational exercise offers important opportunities for socialisation. It also permits the emotional benefits of socially acceptable touching, unconnected with dependence and the need for personal care, a rarity for many long-bereaved, elderly people.

Providing guidance and opportunity

Any exercise programme to improve general fitness must include activities to develop strength, endurance, flexibility, and coordination in a progressive, balanced, and enjoyable way. It must use all major muscle groups in exercises that train through each individual's fullest possible ranges of movement. An exercise programme for older people must also aim to load the bones, target postural and pelvic floor muscles, include practice of functional movements, and emphasise the development of body awareness and balance skills. A combination of regular, recreational brisk walking and swimming, preferably combined with specific exercises to improve strength and flexibility, will meet most of these criteria for most people. Many older people also welcome the opportunity to participate in an exercise group or class.

How much is enough?

Until very recently, published guidelines have recommended vigorous physical activity to achieve the expected benefits to health. There is now ample evidence that substantial health benefits can be obtained by an approach that is more temperate and, arguably, more likely to be sustained. The approach is based on physical activity of moderate intensity, i.e. it makes the participant feel warm and breathe a little more heavily. For most people this is equivalent to the **effort** of brisk walking (although, of course, the **speed** of brisk walking will vary considerably from person to person.) The "message" now is simply "More people, more active, more often".

The older and/or frailer the participant, the greater the potential benefit from the inclusion of strengthening, stretching, balance, and coordination activities.

Exercise classes

A short chapter cannot teach how a seniors' exercise class should be run. Instead, we offer guidance to health professionals on areas to consider when they assess an exercise class to which they might refer patients, or when they seek specialist training to enable them to conduct such classes safely and successfully.

All sessions should start and finish gradually. The warm-up loosens joints, stretches muscles, rehearses skills and gradually increases demand on the heart and lungs. Afterwards, the warm-down consists principally of slow, rhythmic exercises to preserve venous return as muscle and skin vasodilation gradually return to resting levels. It may also incorporate relaxation, held stretches, additional strengthening, and fall management activities in sitting or lying positions.

Many of the activities should be closely related to life and to maintaining independence. Techniques of lifting, walking, and transferring (moving from sitting to standing, standing to lying, even crawling, etc.) should be specifically taught and discussed. Information about the specific benefits of particular exercises is greatly appreciated, for example, shoulder mobility for doing up zips, stamina for "energy" and less breathlessness during

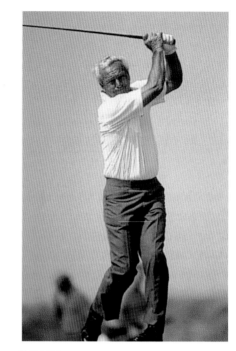

Figure 11.1

At any age:

- 30 minutes of at least moderate intensity physical activity on at least 5 days a week will significantly improve health

- Two 15 minute periods of moderate activity in a day can be beneficial and a good way to begin

- Every little counts towards the 30 minutes activity total. To begin with, if 15 minutes sounds too much, take a 'little-and-often' approach, advising the participant to progress steadily from just 3 minutes, until 3 minutes becomes 5 minutes, then 5 minutes twice a day, increasing to 10, 15 and, finally, 30 minutes of moderate activity

- Maximum benefit to health will probably be gained with 20 minutes of vigorous endurance activity 3 times per week, plus 20 minutes of strengthening twice a week, plus daily stretching, balance, and coordination activities

- Any activity is better than none and even once a week is better than nothing. It's never too late to start. It is best to select enjoyable activities

---

Implications of running 'Fitness for Seniors' classes — I

For the teacher

- Emphasise posture and technique
- Give more teaching points and repeat more often
- Give more warning of directional and step changes
- Improve own body language and demonstration skills
- Improve own observation, monitoring, and correction skills
- Offer more choices
- Offer more information
- Be polished and punctual

exertion, or quadriceps, handgrip, and biceps strength for lifting the holiday suitcase.

Above all, fitness must be fun. Important factors can be the use of appropriate equipment, games, music, and opportunities for socialising (but beware of ageist assumptions about what is appropriate).

Programming

The aim is a long-term commitment to a mixture of activities. The combinations must be tailored to individual health and fitness levels, tastes, interests, and means. They might include walking, swimming, weight-, circuit- or step-training, exercise to music, dancing, chair work, tai chi, tennis, bowls, etc. A home exercise programme can usefully complement the organised sessions. Provision must be made for a wide range of initial levels of habitual physical activity and for a variety of disabilities.

Programmes should provide opportunities for both exclusive seniors' sessions and integration with other age groups for selected activities. Opportunities to socialise should be scheduled at all activities. Year-round programming is essential. Off-peak timing improves use of resources, but must not exclude the many older people still in employment. Teachers should be qualified (see "Education and Training") and must be paid accordingly, but concessionary rates and discretionary financial assistance may be considered for individual participants.

Participants must be involved in planning, selecting and evaluating the programme. The setting should be elder-friendly in respect of public transport, parking, access, ambience, ventilation, lighting, refreshments, changing and toilet facilities, floor surfaces. Thought should be given for those with a disability (for example, stair rails, large print notices, wheelchair access). Promotional material should feature appropriate older role models.

Safety

Injury prevention is a high priority. Even stiffness and minor overuse injuries reduce enjoyment and adherence and can often be avoided. An adequate warm-up, the selection of safe exercises and movement patterns, and regular monitoring of body alignment and exercise intensity are important. Precise, audible teaching instructions and visible, skilled demonstrations are essential. Skillful class management and observation are needed to ensure safety in seniors' fitness sessions. These issues are all taught in specialist courses for those training to run exercise classes for older people. Competence to run such classes (see "Education and Training") implies both theoretical knowledge and practical experience in selecting and supervising safe, appropriate exercises according to the participants' particular medical problems, for example, unsteadiness, breathlessness, angina, arthritis, osteoporosis, or inability to stand.

Opinion is divided over the place of informed consent forms and medical release forms for older adults embarking on unaccustomed physical activity. On the one hand, there is the need to do everything possible to minimise any potential hazard, coupled with a belief that medical review will contribute usefully. On the other hand, there are legitimate concerns about overmedicalisation of recreational activities and the impossibility of detecting all potentially important pathologies. Furthermore, there has been a tendency for medical review to ensure "safety" by exclusion, failing to recognise that those people identified as carrying a risk of adverse events during physical activity are the very ones who stand to gain most by participation (for example, a hypertensive person with diabetes). Fortunately, things are changing and the need is recognised for an "enabling",

> **Implications of running "Fitness for Seniors" classes — II**
>
> **For programming**
> - Include seniors
>   – in planning and staffing
>   – in evaluation
>   – in promotional material
> - Pre-exercise review of health information and functional needs
> - First session is an individual assessment
> - Individualised or tailored programmes
> - Progressive and multi-level programmes
> - Mixture of activities
> - Ensure essential facilities
> - Appropriate scheduling and costing
> - Include socialisation time
> - Include educational opportunities

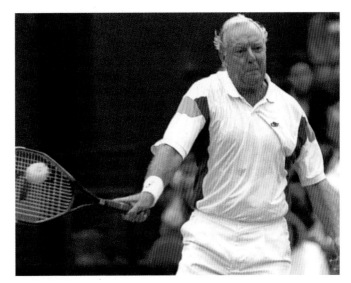

Figure 11.2 A player in the 45 and over tournament at Wimbledon

pre-exercise, medical review, i.e. one that will facilitate safe and effective recreational participation by all older people.

What, then, should doctors do, especially as they will usually be less knowledgeable than the specialist exercise teacher to advise on the individualised prescription of particular exercises or activities? The doctor has three responsibilities. First, to identify the pathologies that are present and to ensure that they and all medications are accurately communicated to the exercise teacher. Second, to highlight any ways they consider the safe conduct of exercise might be influenced by the diagnoses (for example, susceptibility to angina, shortness of breath, arrhythmias, joint pain, confusion etc.) or by any of the medications (for example, by suppressing pain, by producing a bradycardia unrepresentative of exercise intensity, by increasing susceptibility to postural hypotension, etc., *Figure 11.3*).

The doctor's third responsibility is to educate the exercise pupil in the early recognition of symptoms that might indicate the exercise programme was, in some way, unsuitable for them and their particular chronic pathologies. For example, the patient with osteoarthritic knees should be taught to recognise and respect an increase in pain, stiffness, or swelling. The patient with a history of mild, controlled heart failure should be taught that increased breathing during exercise is normal, but that a decrease in the level of exercise required to provoke shortness of breath is abnormal.

Thus, clinical responsibility rests with the referrer. On the other hand, responsibility for the administration, design, and delivery of the programme rests with the leisure management and instructor team and/or the exercise practitioner service (*Figure 11.4*). To take this share of the overall responsibility, those supervising the conduct of the exercise must be able to demonstrate that they have been appropriately trained.

Education and training

In many respects an elderly person is like an athlete; both often perform near their limits. The coaching skills required to ensure both optimal performance and safety are important and specialised.

Exercise England, the English national governing body for exercise and fitness, runs a national registration scheme. Teachers/instructors who are registered are properly qualified and insured, and work to a code of ethics and professional practice. Similar registration schemes are run by Fitness Scotland and Fitness Wales. We recommend that health professionals refer older people only to registered teachers/instructors with specialist qualifications.

The education and training of exercise and fitness teachers in the UK is undergoing considerable change. National occupational standards (NOS) now exist, which describe the knowledge base and practical competencies that exercise and fitness teachers must possess. The teaching of exercise and fitness to older adults is sited at Level 3, the more advanced level of qualification. At this level, requirements include the ability to develop long-term physical activity programmes adapted to accommodate the heterogeneity and the physical limitations of older people. This will require knowledge of the ways in which ageing and medical conditions may affect exercise performance and participation. It is anticipated that these new Level 3 NOS and qualifications will apply from mid 1999. Currently, those teaching this age group can obtain exercise and fitness qualifications through the YMCA Fitness Industry Training and the American College of Sports Medicine, and movement qualifications through the Extend and Excel 2000 organisations. From mid 1999, organisations working in this specialist field will

Figure 11.3 Extract from an Exercise Referral form used by health professionals to transfer clinical information meaningfully to the exercise practitioner (Dinan, Young, Iliffe and Wallace, unpublished)

Figure 11.4 Proforma used by the referring doctor to acknowledge receipt of the exercise practitioner's proposals for an individual patient's Activity Plan (Dinan, Young, Iliffe and Wallace, unpublished)

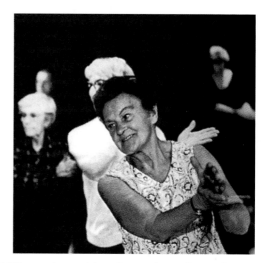

Figure 11.5 The use of appropriate music can make exercise more fun

need to align their education and training to the new NOS at Level 3.

Summary

Physical activity is an important therapeutic and preventive option for middle-aged and older patients. Health professionals are well placed to endorse the "Use it or lose it" message and to give the advice and authoritative encouragement an older person may need to begin or to return to physical recreation. We welcome the growth of exercise referral schemes and urge other health professionals in primary and secondary care to develop close working partnerships with exercise and fitness professionals and with the management of local recreational facilities. Such schemes are popular with primary care professionals, service commissioners, leisure centre managers, instructors, and patients. Their continuing growth will now be supported by national policy guidelines for quality assurance that have been developed in response to a commission from the Department of Health.

Finally, do remember that your own example (as an active person) will have a positive impact on your patients' behaviour!

Acknowledgements

We thank Annette Burgess and Andrew Craig (both of Exercise England) for their assistance in describing developments in training and education. We also thank our collaborators Steve Iliffe and Paul Wallace for permission to include Figures 11.3 and 11.4.

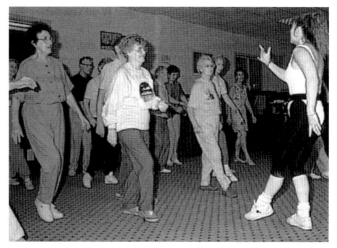
Figure 11.6 Exercise should be safe and well-monitored

Useful contacts

Training and education
National vocational awarding bodies
SNVQ, Edexcel Central House, Upper Woburn Place, London WC1H OHH, Tel: 0171-413-8400

SNVQ, City & Guilds of London Institute, 1 Giltspur Street, London EClA 9DD, Tel: 0171-294-2468

Royal Society of Arts (RSA Examinations Board), Progress House, Westwood Way, Coventry CV4 8HS Tel: 01203-470033

SQA, Hanover House, 24 Douglas Street, Glasgow G2 7NP Tel: 0141-248-7900

SPRITO, The Industry Training Organisation for Sport and Recreation, 24 Stephenson Way, London NI 2HD, Tel: 0171-388-7755

National governing bodies
Exercise England, The English National Governing Body for Exercise & Fitness, Solecast House, 13–27 Brunswick Place, London NI 6DX

Fitness Scotland, Caledonia House, South Gyle, Edinburgh EH12 9DQ, Tel: 0131-317-7243

Fitness Wales, Whitechurch Road, Cardiff CF4 3ND Tel: 01222 520130

Fitness Northern Ireland, 147 Holywood Road, Belfast BT4 3BE, Tel: 01232 651103

Sports Councils
Sport England, 16 Upper Woburn Place, London WC1H OQB, Tel: 0171-273-1500

Sport Scotland, Caledonia House, South Gyle, Edinburgh EH12 9DQ, Tel: 0131-317-7200

Sports Council for Wales, Welsh Institute of Sport, Sophia Gardens, Cardiff CFl 9SN, Tel: 01222-300500

Sports Council for Northern Ireland, House of Sport, Upper Malone Road, Belfast BT9 5LA, Tel: 01232-381222

Training organisations
YMCA Fitness Industry Training, 112 Great Russell Street, London WC1B 3NQ, 0171-343-1850 (Also regional centres throughout UK)

Extend, 22 Maltings Drive, Wheathampstead, Herts AL4 8QJ Tel: 01582-832760

Excel 2000, 1a North Street, Sherringham, Norfolk NR26 8LW, Tel: 01263-825670

Agencies
Age Concern England, (Ageing Well), (Age Resource), Astral House, 1268 London Road, Norbury, London SW16 4ER, Tel: 0181-765-7200

Age Concern Scotland, 54a Fountainbridge, Edinburgh EH3 9PT, Tel: 0131-228-5656

Age Concern Wales, 4th Floor, 1 Cathedral Road Cardiff CFl 9SD, Tel: 01222-371566

Age Concern Northern Ireland, 3 Lower Crescent, Belfast BT7 1NR, Tel: 01232-245729

Association of Retired Persons, Greencourt House, Frances Street, London SW1P 1D2, Tel: 0171-895-8880

Help the Aged, (Sportage), St. James Walk, London EC1R OBE Tel: 0171-253-0253

Ramblers Association, 1/5 Wandsworth Road, London SW8 2XX, Tel: 0171-582-6878

Senior friendly multipurpose fitness equipment

Davies, The Sports People, (Nottingham Rehabilitation Equipment), 1 Ludlow Hill Road, West Bridgford, Nottingham NG2 6HD Tel: 01602-452345

Powersport International Ltd, (Integra Range of Resistance Training Equipment), Queens Road, Bridgend Industrial Estate, Bridgend, Mid Glamorgan, CF31 3UE Tel: 01656-661164

12 Water sports

J D M Douglas

Supervised training and instruction are the essence of safety for water sports. All outdoor adventure sports have predictable risks and survival techniques are best learned through clubs affiliated to their national organisations, such as the British Sub Aqua Club, Royal Yachting Association, British Canoe Union, Royal Yachting Association, and British Water Ski Federation. They produce statistics based on accident reports and modify training procedures if trends are noted. They all have honorary medical support.

Swimming

Benefits and contraindications
Swimming is a physical activity that can be enjoyed safely by people at any age. Gentle swimming provides an injury-free method of exercising joints and muscles. It is the ideal exercise to prevent and rehabilitate musculoskeletal injuries to the neck and back. Breast stroke requires repeat flexion and extension of the neck, whereas front crawl develops erector spinae, psoas, and latissimus dorsi. Patients with paraplegia gain confidence from the buoyancy given to weak limbs.

People who have had hip or knee replacements should avoid breast stroke because the frog leg kick risks dislocation. Those with multiple joint replacements should be advised that they may be negatively buoyant.

Antenatal water exercise
"Aqua-natal" classes are a new fashion in antenatal care, which should be encouraged and supported by doctors. Trained midwives supervise "water aerobics" to music while the pregnant women stand in a pool and use floating for relaxation. Participation can be encouraged (in swimmers and non-swimmers) from the first trimester to near term to help posture and breathing in a "weightless" environment. Postnatally, babies can be reintroduced to swimming with care for their temperature from about 3 months. Children with grommets may swim on the surface from one month after insertion at the surgeon's discretion.

Oxygen uptake with different strokes
Comparative studies of oxygen uptake in triathletes suggest that speed is related to skill rather than aerobic power. The oxygen cost of swimming at a constant speed differs with strokes, front crawl being the most energy efficient.

Cardiovascular fitness
Swimming improves cardiovascular fitness for healthy people, but needs to be regular and vigorous; 20 minutes continuous swimming, three times a week, is ideal. A swimmer of average ability should be able to cover half a mile (32 lengths of a 25 metre pool) without stopping.

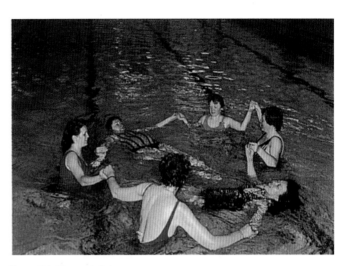

Figure 12.1 "Aqua-natal" class

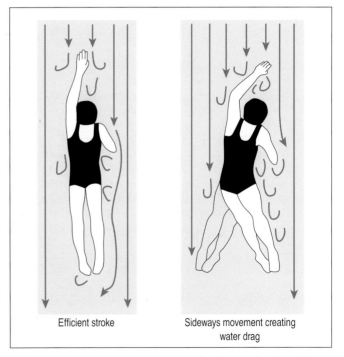

Efficient stroke | Sideways movement creating water drag

Figure 12.2 Swimming efficiency and front crawl: left—efficient stroke; right—sideways movement creating water drag

Cardiac rehabilitation

Heart rates during swimming are lower than during equivalent land-based exercise, and venous return is encouraged by hydrostatic pressure. Patients can be encouraged to return to swimming six to eight weeks after myocardial infarction.

Special problems in competitive swimmers

Chlorine conjunctivitis

This can be prevented by wearing good goggles. Chronic otitis externa caused by bacterial or fungal infection in the macerated external ear canal can be treated topically with ear drops. Some swimmers find prophylactic alcohol and acetic acid drops or ear plugs helpful. Bony exostosis of the external auditory meatus may require surgical removal.

Shoulder pain

Front crawl and butterfly stroke cause shoulder pain by repeated abduction followed by forced adduction. This movement requires the rotator cuff muscles to pull the humeral head under the acromium, which may result in subacromial bursitis or impingement syndrome. Treatment is rest with nonsteroidal anti-inflammatory drugs or steroid injections into the subacromial bursa. The shoulder joint becomes unstable in back crawl and may partially dislocate with each stroke, which leads to tears of the cartilaginous rim of the glenoid socket. Avoiding using hand paddles and doing exercises to strengthen the rotator cuff muscles will help prevent this problem.

Knee pain

Knee pain in breast stroke results from the repeated valgus forces on the knee putting a strain on the medial collateral ligament. Flexion and extension of the knee in all strokes can cause patella compression pain and chondromalacia patella. Quadriceps exercise and using neoprene knee braces during training may help.

Immersion and drowning

Low water temperature

Outdoor water sports in the United Kingdom inland and coastal waters require planning to deal with voluntary or involuntary immersion in water from 0°C to 12°C. The thermal conductivity of water is 20 times that of air and cooling occurs over time in water temperatures below 34°C. In cold water, the body's outer shell attempts to protect the inner core temperature by peripheral vasoconstriction in the limbs, making them feel useless. Normal deep body temperature is 37°C; mental confusion, sleepiness, and loss of will to survive develop at 34°C core temperature. Unconsciousness at 30°C and ventricular fibrillation below 28°C lead to death at around 24°C.

Hypothermia

Channel swimmers survive because of their fat distribution. Adolescents seem to be particularly vulnerable to cold stress in water or on mountains because of their large surface area in proportion to their low body volume. Early symptoms of hypothermia include apathy and withdrawal. Sudden immersion in icecold water quickly incapacitates even very strong swimmers, with reflex tachycardia, hypertension, and hyperventilation sometimes leading to sudden death.

Long distance swimming competitions in fresh or sea water need careful safety and contingency planning with the assistance of a doctor who understands hypothermia physiology. Young

Comparative oxygen uptake and heart rate in the same swimmer using different strokes at constant speed

Stroke	Speed (m/s)	Oxygen uptake (l/min)	Heart rate (beats/min)
Front crawl	1.0	1.83	125
Backstroke	1.0	2.42	138
Butterfly	1.0	2.85	150
Breast stroke	1.0	3.42	162

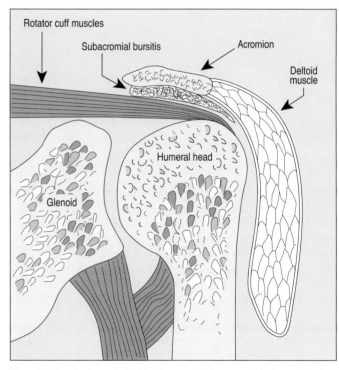

Figure 12.3 Crawl swimmers' shoulder. Repeated impingement of the humeral head into the overlying acromion

Thermal protection

- Neoprene wet suits are worn in most water sports during the summer months throughout the UK and can increase survival times by up to 24 hours. An outer windproof shell garment increases their efficiency

- Dry suits are waterproof "bags" sealed at the neck and wrists. Thermal underclothing increases their efficiency for winter water sports, but they lose their buoyancy if punctured

- Survival advice for sailors in the water includes staying with the boat and, to conserve heat, adopting a fetal position and not swimming

- In boats, people should lie down to avoid wind chill and give priority to insulating the head and neck, as these are the areas of greatest heat loss once the circulation has adapted to cold stress

- Alcohol consumption is strongly associated with deaths from drowning and with cervical spine injuries resulting from diving into shallow water. It also potentiates cold stress by vasodilatation, hypoglycaemia and mental confusion

adult males will be at particular risk even if they are excellent pool swimmers. A rowing boat or canoe should be allocated to each competitor with a remit to observe and signal to a fast inflatable rescue boat in case of difficulty with the swimmer. Pulling a distressed, slippery swimmer into a rowing boat is impractical. Planning to rescue several swimmers at once in deteriorating sea conditions requires at least one inflatable rescue boat for four swimmers, as outboard engines may fail and distance to and from shore facilities may be lengthy. Large polythene 'mountain type' survival bags should be kept in rescue boats. Collapse and cramp is a common occurrence in the water after profound exertion to cross the finishing line.

Hydrostatic pressure

Immersion exerts a hydrostatic squeeze on venous return. After prolonged immersion (only possible if a life jacket is worn) sudden release of the pressure by lifting the casualty in an upright position may lead to circulatory collapse. Rescue in the supine position is, therefore, recommended, but may be impossible in practice.

Resuscitation

The dilemma for doctors in an outdoor environment is when to start chest compression. Severe hypothermia may produce an impalpable carotid pulse and rough handling may precipitate ventricular fibrillation.

Swallowed or inhaled water

The stomach is usually full of water swallowed during near drowning. No attempt should be made to 'empty the lungs' of water because the volumes aspirated are small. Restoring a heart beat, monitoring cardiac function, and administering high concentration oxygen are essential first aid measures. In hospital, the rectal temperature and an electrocardiogram should be taken before resuscitation is abandoned. Victims of near drowning who have inhaled water should be kept under observation for at least 24 hours in case pulmonary oedema develops.

Fresh or salt water

Management after immersion in fresh water is no different from that after salt water immersion.

Leptospirosis

Stagnant inland water may be contaminated by this spirochaete from rat or cattle urine. The presenting symptom is an illness like influenza that starts 7–12 days after exposure. The haemorrhagic complications of Weil's disease are prevented by early recognition and treatment with penicillin, erythromycin, or tetracycline. Cuts should be covered before immersion and showers taken afterwards. Doctors should be informed of the risk by the sports person.

Sport diving

There are about 70 000 scuba divers in Britain. (Scuba stands for self-contained underwater breathing apparatus.) Each year there are about 12 deaths and 70 episodes of decompression illness that require recompression. These should, however, be set against the several hundred thousand dives, which means that mortality and morbidity compares favourably with those for mountaineering, a sport with similar levels of risk and numbers of devotees.

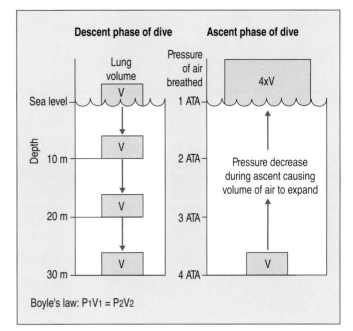

Figure 12.4

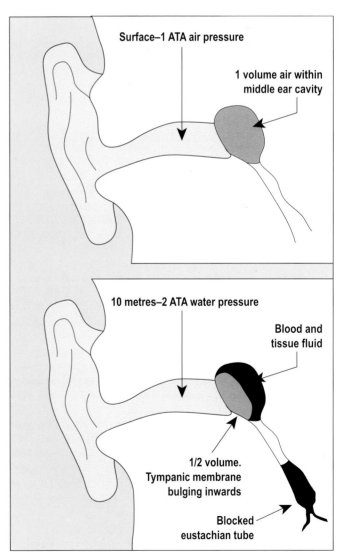

Figure 12.5

Breathing compressed air during descent

To equalise the pressure in the body's air-filled cavities (sinuses, middle ear space, and lungs) divers breathe air from an aqualung at a pressure equal to that of the surrounding water. Water pressure increases by one atmosphere absolute (1 ATA or 1 bar) for every 10 metres of descent and the gases behave according to the physical gas laws.

Blocking of a eustachian tube during descent will lead to aural barotrauma, which is the most common dysbaric illness. Divers should be warned never to force ear clearing by going deeper despite pain. Repeated practice, Valsalva, and ephedrine nasal drops prior to diving may help. Excision of Vomero ethmoid suture operations are successful for preventing persisting difficulties. In acute injury, bruising of the tympanic membrane should resolve within two weeks and antibiotics are usually required. Perforations need to be healed completely before diving is resumed. Rarely, the inner ear also becomes damaged, causing an oval or round window perilymph leak. Tinnitus, vertigo, and deafness require urgent assessment by an ear, nose, and throat specialist.

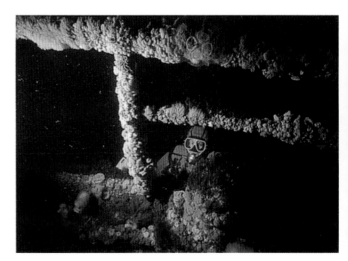

Figure 12.6 Diver at a wreck in UK waters

Nitrogen narcosis

Nitrogen is highly soluble in fat and exerts a narcotic effect on the central nervous system as its partial pressure increases. At depths below 30 metres, nitrogen narcosis has an effect similar to that of alcohol intoxication and is a serious hazard to personal safety. The resulting euphoria, overconfidence, poor mental judgement, and aggravation of panic are potentiated by drugs acting on the central nervous system, which are contraindicated in diving. Nitrogen narcosis resolves spontaneously without any hangover when the diver ascends to a shallower depth. Helium is much less soluble in fat and must be used to replace nitrogen at depths below 50 metres in commercial diving.

Acute decompression illness

The current descriptive, clinical classification of decompression illness makes no attempt to discriminate between the pathophysiological mechanisms of pulmonary barotrauma and decompression sickness used previously.

Air in the lungs must be vented while divers surface because the expansion of gas volume predicted by Boyle's Law will result in pulmonary barotrauma if there is any attempt at breath holding or if a person has an air trapping disease. Cerebral arterial gas embolism, pneumothorax, or mediastinal emphysema can result from an uncontrolled ascent. A diver who becomes unconscious or has the unilateral signs of a cerebrovascular accident after an uncontrolled ascent requires immediate recompression in a chamber to preserve life.

Nitrogen that has dissolved in body tissue during a dive must be excreted via the lungs during the ascent and after surfacing. Bubbles of nitrogen form in the tissues and blood if pressure is reduced too quickly. Gas trapped in soft tissues around a joint gives rise to shoulder or elbow pain and, when more widely disseminated in the body, to chest pains or neurological symptoms. Decompression illness can be reduced, but not eliminated, by using decompression stoppage tables or wrist-held diving computers to control ascents.

Oxygen toxicity occurs on deep diving with 100% oxygen. However, Nitrox breathing mixtures that blend oxygen and nitrogen in different proportions (depending on depth) allow longer bottom times for equivalent air depths. Trimix, using helium, nitrogen, and oxygen mixtures facilitates very deep scuba diving, but the risks are substantially increased.

Neurological symptoms occurring within 24 hours of surfacing must be considered to be a manifestation of acute

Acute decompression illness

Forms of onset	Manifestations
Progressive	Cutaneous
Static	Neurological
Relapsing	Cardiopulmonary
Spontaneous	Joint pain
	Constitutional

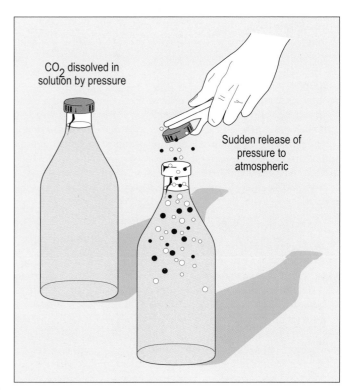

CO_2 dissolved in solution by pressure

Sudden release of pressure to atmospheric

Figure 12.7 Solubility of gases in liquids

decompression illness until proved otherwise. They must be treated urgently by recompression. Divers will usually describe chest pains within 10 minutes of surfacing; these resolve, but proceed to a deep, boring, lumbar backache and girdle pains. Loss of feeling, motor power, and coordination of the legs can quickly proceed to permanent spinal paralysis. A diver who cannot walk or pass urine when in an accident and emergency department requires 100% oxygen and immediate transfer to a hyperbaric unit for recompression, after liaison with the unit about the means of transport. Air transport is quick, but altitude causes the bubbles to expand. Indeed, decompression illness may initially manifest itself after a flight home from a foreign diving holiday.

Diving safety

Medical examinations
The United Kingdom Sport Diving Medical Committee (C/O BSAC Headquarters, Telfords Quay, Ellesmere Port, Cheshire L45 4FY) requires people to have a thorough medical examination before starting training with a club. This committee is an international source of experience and advice for evidence-based recommendations on sport diving medical standards. The examination forms contain guidance for the doctor and lists of voluntary medical referees to consult in doubtful cases.

Chronic illnesses
Improvement in the treatment and self-monitoring of diabetes and asthma has allowed the United Kingdom club to select and train people with these conditions when previous advice has been to ban such participants. However, epilepsy and drugs acting on the central nervous system are usually contraindications to sport diving. There are schemes to make diving a sport that is inclusive for people with disabilities through special training and organisations. (The Dolphin Network, C/O Diving Diseases Research Centre, Taymor Science Park, Derreford, Plymouth). The risk assessment for individuals with chronic illnesses needs expert advice from medical referees because diver rescues can put other lives at risk.

Training
Good basic training within a recognised club or training organisation remains the cornerstone of diving safety.

Other water sports

Canoeing
Helmets are required in white water canoeing because head injury is an obvious risk. Anterior dislocation of the shoulder can be caused by extreme high brace manoeuvres. Wrist tenosynovitis can occur in long-distance kayaking, but is prevented by cranked paddle handles and angled blades.

Sailing and board sailing
Competitive dinghy and board sailing required prolonged tension in the abdominal, quadriceps, and back leg muscles to balance the wind forces. Anterior knee pain can also occur in

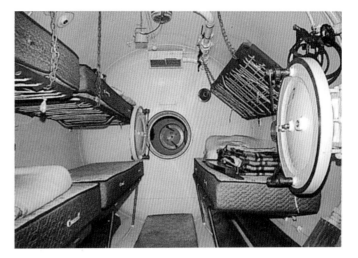

Figure 12.8 Inside of a recompression chamber

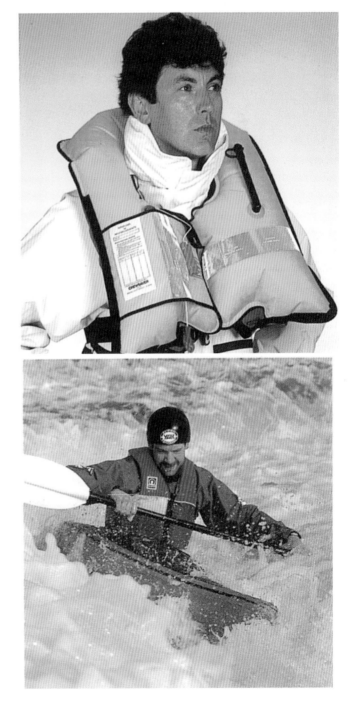

Figure 12.9 A new European standard specifies the correct choice of life jacket or buoyancy aid for different applications. **Top**: a life jacket must self-right an unconscious non-swimmer but may be uncomfortable to wear or require the maintenance of CO_2 cylinders. **Bottom**: buoyancy aids are a safe alternative, giving freedom of movement during sport and once immersed. Wet suits are also buoyant

young dinghy sailors with chondromalacia patellas. Standing in the wind, repeated immersion and exertion make board sailors at risk of exhaustion and hypothermia.

In yachts, an unexpected movement of the main sail (involuntary gybe) may cause serious head injury or sweep a sailor overboard. Clothing, safety lines, and life jackets should be planned in advance of changing weather conditions. Cold stress is serious in combination with prolonged seasickness; cinnarazine tablets or hyoscine patches are popular prophylactic measures against seasickness.

Water skiing
Propeller and impact injuries are an obvious risk, but can be prevented by following boat safety procedures and by wearing helmets for ski jumping. Serious injury has been caused by water douching into the vagina or rectum during ski jumping, but this can be prevented by wearing a wet suit.

Rowing
Rowing is a safe sport with a low injury rate, but it can cause low back pain and tenosynovitis of the wrist.

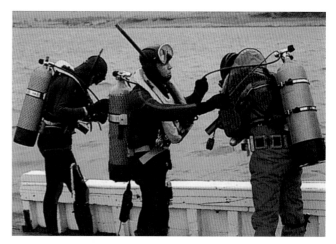

Figure 12.10 Safety relies on diving in pairs

Summary

- Swimming can be advocated as a safe exercise to maintain physical fitness and aid rehabilitation from *in utero* to old age
- Alcohol is associated with deaths in all watersports
- Hypothermia needs to be anticipated and prevented in all outdoor watersports
- Inland watersports risk *leptospirosis*. Participants and doctors need to remember this unusual, but treatable illness to prevent fatalities
- Neurological symptoms occurring within 24 hours of a scuba dive are a medical emergency requiring expert advice and recompression treatment. Oxygen and fluids should be given during transport to the chamber.

Further reading

British Sub Aqua Club Diving Manual. British Sub-Aqua Club, Telfords Quay, Ellesmere Port, Cheshire L65 4FY

Costhill D (1991) S*wimming: Handbook of Sports Medicine and Science*, IOC Series. Blackwell Scientific Publications, Oxford

Edmonds C, Lowrie C, Pennefather J, eds (1992) *Diving and Subaquatic Medicine*. Butterworth Heinemann, Oxford

Acknowledgements

The table showing oxygen uptake with different swimming strokes and the drawings showing efficiency of front crawl and crawl swimmers' shoulder are reproduced with permission from Blackwell Scientific Publications.

Emergency phone numbers for diving emergencies
- HM Coastguard (via 999 or VHF Channel 16) provide communication links for all maritime emergencies

England and Wales:
- Royal Navy: 01831 151523
- Plymouth area: 01752 261910

Scotland:
- Aberdeen: 01224 681818

Ireland:
- Craigavon: 01762 336711

13 Sport and disability

A D J Webborn

Despite the fact that the Paralympic Games is now the world's second largest sporting event after the Olympic Games in terms of numbers of competitors, the achievements of athletes with disabilities have remained largely unknown to the majority. A high jump of nearly two metres by a single leg amputee or sub one hour thirty minutes for the wheelchair marathon show that people with disabilities are capable of considerable athletic performance. It is important that these achievements should be recognised by the medical profession for two major reasons. First, that these people are athletes in their own right who have their own sports medicine needs. Secondly, to help alter their attitudes to patients with disabilities in relation to physical activity, where many doctors are restrictive rather than prescriptive with exercise.

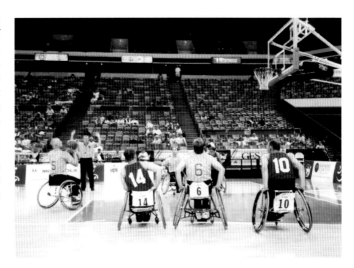

Figure 13.1 Wheelchair basketball, Atlanta 1996, Aus v. GB

General health

The beneficial effects of exercise are well established in relation to general health and in regard to prevention and/or management of specific disease processes (for example non-insulin dependent diabetes). People with physical disabilities are less likely to avail themselves of these benefits for a variety of reasons, including cultural and social factors, facilities, and access. Participation in sport is not essential, but it is important that people with disabilities are encouraged to remain physically active. The same message of accumulation of, at least, 30 minutes of moderate intensity activity on, at least, five days of the week is equally applicable to someone with a disability. The principles of training, i.e. the graded increase in duration, intensity, and frequency of activity, also apply, but more thought may be required as to the mode of exercise according to the disability. The social and psychological benefits of exercise and sport participation are not exclusive to the able-bodied and there can be major improvements in self-esteem and social integration through an active lifestyle.

Choosing an activity or sport

In reality, people with disabilities can take part in virtually every sport available, including high-risk sports, such as mountain climbing, sub-aqua diving, and skiing. Some sports are conventional sports in which little or no modification is required, for example, swimming. Other sports may require specific adaptation, for example, wheelchair basketball, or may be specifically developed for a certain disability, such as goalball for the visually impaired. For those who are counselling people with disabilities about the potential benefits of sport, it is important to establish their aims. If the aim is primarily for physical health benefits for a general health or disease modification, then one has to consider the difference between exercise and sport. These

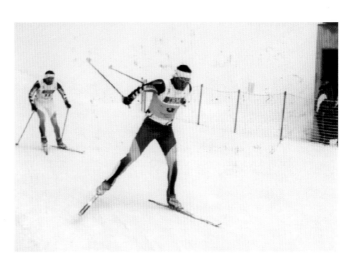

Figure 13.2: Guide leading visually impaired skier; Cross country, Nagano 1998

terms are often used interchangeably and incorrectly. Sport is not always exercise and vice versa. Sport implies competition and the physiological demands are determined by the sport, for example wheelchair sprint racing (anaerobic) versus wheelchair road racing (aerobic) versus pistol shooting (skill). Sport may also involve trauma, which is particularly undesirable in some conditions. Alternatively, the focus may be on socialisation and building self-esteem. While the ability to achieve one of these aims is not necessarily exclusive of the others, it is helpful to consider one's goals. Not all sports need to be organised or competitive. The choice of sport will be influenced by various factors, including:

- The personal preference of the person—an emphasis on enjoyment and participation in a sport that stimulates the person may be important for continued participation
- The characteristics of the sport—physiological demands, collision potential, team or individual co-ordination requirements
- The medical condition—beneficial and detrimental aspects
- Conditions associated with the condition-—although motor dysfunction may initially appear to be the major limitation to participation, there may be, for example, an associated cardiac condition to consider
- The cognitive ability and social skills of the person—ability to follow rules and interact with others
- Availability of facilities
- Availability of appropriate coaching and support staff (for example, lifting and handling)
- Equipment availability and cost—as disability sport has evolved, so has the technology. Specialist chairs are available for sports such as tennis, rugby, and basketball. While it is not necessary to have sport-specific chairs for initial participation, it does become a consideration as people develop their interest and feel more limited by their equipment.

Risks of participation

In general terms, there are relatively few absolute contra-indications to participation in physical activity for people, whether or not they are able-bodied, if the general training principles of gradual and progressive overload are applied.

Risks to consider
- Cardiac conditions
- Environmental factors
- Trauma
- Overuse injuries

Cardiac conditions
Sudden deaths associated with vigorous exercise or sports participation, are predominantly related to cardiac conditions. For people with a disability, their physician needs greater awareness of conditions that may have associated cardiac disease. Exercise intensity is an important consideration in sport selection where cardiac anomalies may be present ,for example Down's syndrome

Environmental factors
Risks of heat or cold injury may occur due to loss of autonomic function in, for example, spinal cord injury. Bilateral leg

---

Factors to consider when choosing a sport
- Personal preference
- Medical condition
- Physiological demands
- Coordination requirements
- Collision potential
- Facilities, equipment, coaching, and support staff
- Team or individual
- Cognitive and social skills

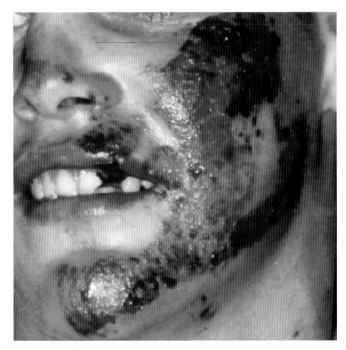

Figure 13.3 Collision potential — cycling

amputees will have reduced surface area for evaporative cooling during exercise in a hot environment

Trauma
Sport may be classified by risk of collision potential, for example skiing or cycling, or it may be a contact sport, such as football. Bone mineral density may be reduced by the nature of the condition, for example, osteogenesis imperfecta, or secondary to immobilisation, for example, in paraplegia, and the risk of spontaneous fracture or fracture with minimal trauma exists. The risk of atlanto-axial instability in people with Down's syndrome remains an issue of contention

Overuse injuries
The potential for overuse injury occurs in any athlete in regular training, but there are certain predisposing factors that are likely to be more prevalent:

- Biomechanical factors—gait in cerebral palsy, or scoliosis in spina bifida
- Technical factors—co-ordination difficulties or restriction of movement altering correct technique.

History of competitive sport

Although sports associations for people with disabilities have existed since the nineteenth century, the credit for the evolution of major games for athletes with disabilities is rightly attributed to the vision and efforts of Sir Ludwig Guttmann. Guttmann was a neurosurgeon at the spinal injuries unit at Stoke Mandeville Hospital near Aylesbury, in England who introduced sport as part of the rehabilitation programme of his patients. Guttman believed that "by restoring activity of mind and body—by instilling self-respect, self-discipline, a competitive spirit, and comradeship—sport develops mental attitudes that are essential for social reintegration". The competitive spirit resulted in an archery competition on the front lawns of the hospital between 16 wheelchair competitors from the spinal unit and a disabled ex-serviceman's home in London. This was in July 1948 on the opening day of the Olympic Games in London and the start of the first Stoke Mandeville Games. In the Sydney Paralympic Games in 2000, they expect to host more than 5000 competitors from six major disability groups (see 1–6 below). Historically sports for people with disabilities have developed in certain sports for certain disabled groups.

1 Spinal cord lesions, congenital (spina bifida) or acquired (injury or disease)

2 Visually impaired

3 Cerebral palsy

4 Amputees

5 "Les Autres"—or "the others" is a term used for people with certain disabilities that do not fit into another category, for example, muscular dystrophy, or multiple sclerosis

6 Learning difficulties

7 Hearing impaired—the deaf still maintain their own organisation, the Comité International Sports des Sourds (CISS) and games (the Silent Games).

To produce fair competition, athletes are placed into different classifications according to their disability. Some sports are restricted to certain disability groups, for example, judo for the visually impaired. Others allow cross-disability competition by functional assessment of sport performance as well as objective assessment by medical examination, for example, in swimming.

Sports of the 1996 Paralympic Games

Archery	Athletics	Basketball	Boccia	Cycling
Equestrian	Fencing	Football	Goalball	Judo
Lawn bowls	Powerlifiting	Shooting	Swimming	Table tennis
Tennis	Volleyball	Yachting	Quad rugby	

Sports of the 1998 Winter Paralympic Games

Alpine skiing

Nordic skiing including biathlon

Sledge racing

Sledge hockey

Paralympic disability groups

1 Spinal cord lesions

2 Visually impaired

3 Cerebral palsy

4 Amputees

5 "Les Autres"

6 Learning difficulties

Medical issues relating to the disability groups

Spinal cord lesions

The motor loss that occurs following spinal cord injury reflects the level of the lesion but several other factors should be considered:

- Loss of intercostal muscle function with reduced ventilatory capacity

- Postural stability, scoliosis may require bracing for some sports

- Sensory loss—skin pressure: increased pressure and shear forces from sports activities may increase the risk of skin ulceration

- Autonomic impairment
  - *Bowels and bladder*—it is important that dehydration does not occur as this not only impairs sport performance and risks heat illness, but is also likely to aggravate renal calculi and infection
  - *Thermal regulation*—loss of peripheral receptor mechanism, control of the sweating effector mechanism, and control of the ability to appropriately vasoconstrict or vasodilate the peripheral vasculature. In the cold environment, the muscles will not shiver, and the skin responses are not appropriate and increase the rate of heat loss
  - *Cardiovascular*—a spinal cord lesion above the level of T1 will cause an absence of sympathetic cardiac innervation producing a depressed maximal heart rate; the level is determined by the intrinsic sinoatrial activity (110–130 beats per minute)
  - *Autonomic dysreflexia*—an inappropriate response triggered by nociceptive input below the level of the lesion producing hypertension, sweating, skin blotching, and headache. The usual causes are blockage of a urinary catheter, constipation, urinary calculi, anal fissure, or in-growing toenail. It can produce severe hypertension, cerebral haemorrhage, fits, and death and, as such, is treated as a medical emergency with treatment aimed at removing the nociceptive stimulus and reduction of blood pressure with sublingual nifedipine. There have been reports of athletes with a quadriplegia

intentionally inducing the dysreflexic state to achieve performance enhancement. This technique is known as "boosting" and has produced increases in simulated race times of 9.7%. It has been deemed a banned method of doping by the International Paralympic Committee

– *Musculoskeletal injuries*—data on the true incidence and type of injury in people with spinal cord lesions are limited. Chronic and overuse symptoms in the cervical and thoracic spines and the shoulder are not uncommon, as are traumatic injuries to the forearm, hand, and fingers

Spina bifida

Depending on the level of the motor loss, people may be ambulant or require a wheelchair for activity. Those who are ambulant have relatively few limitations in sport. Those with higher lesions are more prone to significant scoliosis that may require bracing or spinal fusion. Contractures are common and stretching and flexibility should be an important part of the exercise programme. Bowel and bladder function and sensory loss may be present, but not the autonomic problems of the spinally injured.

Visually impaired

Visual impairment can range from complete blindness to partial sightedness combining loss of visual acuity and field loss. Adaptations to sports include a sound-emitting ball for goalball or cricket, or a tandem cycle with a sighted pilot rider. In swimming, an assistant taps the head or shoulder of the swimmer with a soft-ended pole to indicate the pool end to enable turning and finishing. Adaptations can be made to rifles to emit an audible tone when on target. The main problems specific to the disability include falls and collisions causing injury

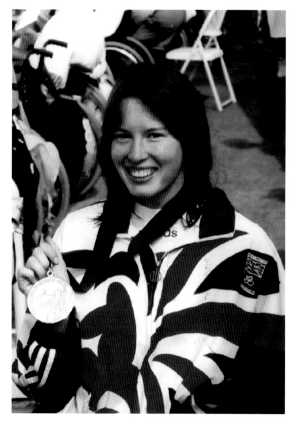

Figure 13.4 "Success"—Jeanette Esling, Swimmer; Atlanta 1996

Cerebral palsy

The three primary motor disorders that are characteristic of the condition are spasticity, choreo-athetosis, or ataxia. Hypotonic cerebral palsy is less common. Commonly associated disorders that should be considered in sport selection include:

• Epilepsy
• Visual defects
• Deafness
• Intellectual impairment
• Perceptual deficits
• Speech impairment

At elite level, 50% of competitors will compete in a wheelchair, while the rest are ambulant.

Amputees

Amputees may participate in sport with a prosthesis (for example, sprinting, cycling) or without (for example, high jump, swimming), or may compete in a wheelchair (for example, basketball). The main risks to the residual limb occur from the effects of friction and compression when a prosthesis is used. Impact loading is also a concern for the residual limb, with increased ground reaction forces that may lead to degenerative change in joints higher in the kinetic chain. Technological

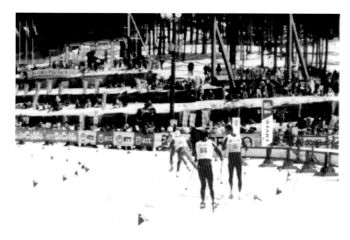

Figure 13.5 Cross country for visually impaired; Nagano 1998

advances in prosthetic design may reduce this loading, while storing energy to facilitate propulsion.

"Les autres"

This term is used to describe those people with certain disabilities that do not fit into another category. Examples include the muscular dystrophies, multiple sclerosis and short stature or limb deficiencies. It is beyond the scope of this text to describe each of these in detail.

Doping issues

The list of banned and permitted substances is the same as the I.O.C., and a few athletes have tested positive for banned substances and received penalties. A far greater proportion of athletes with disabilities will be taking prescribed medication and the attending physician should be aware of this. For sample collection:

- Visually impaired—must be accompanied by an individual to confirm appropriate sample collection is made
- Urine leg bag collection system—the bag must be removed for the collection to be made
- Self-catheterisation—the athletes are allowed to use their own catheter, but the bladder must first be emptied and the sample collected from the next available urine collection.

Summary

The medical care of athletes with disabilities is a challenge for the physician that requires an ability to think laterally. The accepted principles of sports medicine practice need to be re-evaluated in light of the disability of the individual. There is a large void in the scientific research in sport and exercise medicine for people with disabilities that demands further attention, but the achievements of these athletes should inspire us to fill that void.

Further reading

DePauw KP and Gavron SJ (1995) Disability and sport. *Human Kinetics*, Champaign, Ill

Fallon KE (1995) The disabled athlete. In: Bloomfield J, Fricker PA, Fitch KD, eds. *Science and Medicine in Sport*. Blackwell Science, Carlton: 550–51

Goldberg B (1995) Sports and exercise for children with chronic health conditions. *Human Kinetics*, Champaign, Ill

Webborn ADJ (1996) Heat-related problems for the Paralympic Games, Atlanta 1996. *Br J Ther Rehab* **3**: 429–36

> **Doping issues**
> - I.O.C. list of banned substances used
> - Many athletes using prescribed medications
> - Special guidelines for sample collection

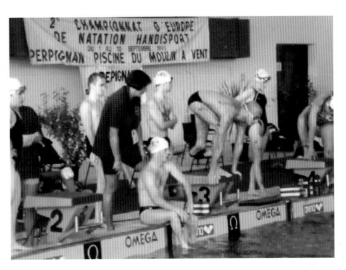

Figure 13.6 "Drinks at the poolside — Swimmers in training" — European Swimming Championships: Perpignan 1995

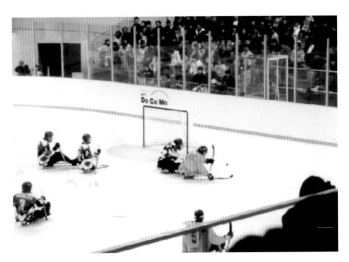

Figure 13.7 Sledge hockey — Nagano 1998

14 Temperature and performance: heat

Thomas Reilly

The environment

The environmental temperature in which athletes have to compete or train is rarely conducive to optimal performance. The athlete may be endangered in extremes of cold (hypothermia) or heat (hyperthermia). Climatic factors to consider are ambient temperature, humidity, radiant heat, air velocity, and precipitation (rain, sleet etc.). The human body gains or loses heat according to prevailing conditions and can modify heat exchange with the environment by appropriate behaviour, such as exercise and choice of clothing.

Despite large fluctuations in environmental conditions, core body temperature is normally maintained within a narrow range about a mean of 37°C. The temperature in the periphery of the body is more variable, but is normally about 4°C below core temperature, thus affecting the gradient for dissipating heat from the internal organs—heart, viscera, and the brain. The size of the gradient between the skin and the environment determines the amount of heat that is lost and gained by the body.

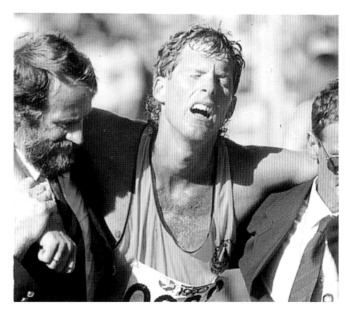

Figure 14.1

Mechanisms of heat exchange

Heat production (gain)	Heat loss
Convection (C)	Evaporation (E)
Radiation (R)	Convection (C)
Conduction (K)	Radiation (R)
Activity	Conduction
Shivering	
Increased basal metabolism	
Basal metabolism	

M–S = E± C±R±K
(M = metabolic heat production, S = storage)

Physiology of thermoregulation

The body generates heat at rest by its metabolic processes. Heat production may be increased 25-fold during strenuous exercise, around 20% contributing to useful work. The remaining 80% is dissipated internally, causing muscle and core temperature to rise.

The first main mechanism for losing heat is by routing more of the cardiac output through the skin where heat is off-loaded from the 'shell' to the environment. Secondly, sweat is secreted on the body's surface where it can evaporate. Evaporation is the main means of losing heat during exercise, but the mechanism is obstructed in high relative humidity when the environment is

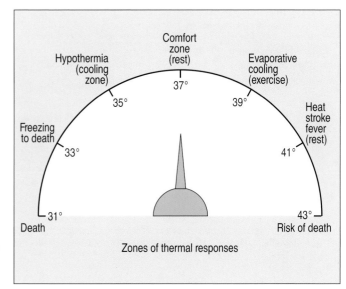

Figure 14.2 The zones of body temperature responses

already highly saturated with water vapour. As cardiac output subserves both thermoregulation and oxygen supply to active muscles, the exercise itself must be lowered to avoid a further rise in core temperature.

Thermoregulatory controls override those of body water regulation, as fluid is lost following stimulation of eccrine sweat glands. Dehydration also leads to a decrement in performance, particularly in events affected by lowered plasma volume. Therefore, progressive fluid loss compounds the consequences of body temperature rising beyond its optimum level.

The temperature of the circulating blood is detected by specialised neurones in the hypothalamus; cells in the anterior portion respond to a temperature rise, cells in the posterior part respond to falling temperature. These areas also receive afferent information from skin receptors about changes in the temperature in the body's immediate environment.

The anterior hypothalamus initiates vasodilation of the skin's circulation when off-loading heat to the environment is required. A balance is effected (largely by the hormones renin and angiotensin) whereby vasodilation does not compromise blood pressure. The sweat glands are activated by sympathetic cholinergic nerve fibres; vasoactive substances from the glands also increase blood flow. Normally, the body acts as a heat sink at the beginning of exercise; sweat droplets appear on the skin's surface after about 7 minutes of exercise at 70% of maximal oxygen uptake.

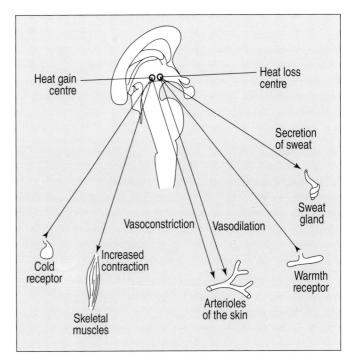

Figure 14.3 Nervous control of temperature regulation

Effects of heat on performance

Elevation of muscle temperature by 1–2°C facilitates performance and reflects the benefit of a pre-competitive warm-up. The consequences of sustaining exercise are the loss of body water associated with sweating and the demands on the circulatory system for thermoregulation. Hypohydration leads to progressive impairment of exercise performance, as indicated by both laboratory-based criteria and field measures. The declines are evident in both cognitive and motor components of performance.

In field games, the activity is intermittent and acyclical, but the high-intensity bouts of exercise are mainly affected. The distance covered in such efforts declines by about 40% at a temperature of 30°C compared to 20°C. Players have to learn to pace their activity levels to suit prevailing conditions and to replace fluid when breaks in play permit. The optimal ambient temperature for marathon running is around 14°C for top runners; this may be too low for those unable to run fast enough to maintain heat balance.

Heat acclimatisation

The main features of heat acclimatisation are an earlier onset of sweating (sweat produced at a lower rise in body temperature) and a more dilute secretion from the sweat glands. Loss of sodium in sweat and urine is reduced due to the action of the hormone aldosterone. The heat-acclimatised individual sweats more than an unacclimatised counterpart at a given exercise intensity. There is also a better distribution of blood to the skin for more effective cooling after a period of acclimatisation, although the acclimatised individual depends more on evaporative sweat loss than on blood flow.

Heat acclimatisation occurs relatively quickly and is practically complete within 10–14 days of the initial exposure. Such adaptations enhance the athlete's capability to perform well under heat stress. Ideally, therefore, the athlete or team should be

Pre-acclimatisation strategies

- The athlete should seek out the hottest time of day to train at home, thus being exposed to the highest heat load available naturally

- If the conditions at home are too cool, an environmental chamber may be used for periodic bouts of heat exposure. It is important to exercise rather than rest under such conditions. About 3 hours per week exercising in an environmental chamber are recommended

- The microclimate next to the skin may be kept hot by wearing heavy sweat suits or windbreakers. This will add to the heat load imposed under cool environmental conditions and induce a degree of adaptation to thermal strain

- Repeated exposure to a sauna or Turkish bath is only partially effective

exposed to the climate of the host country for at least 10 days before the event. An alternative is to have an acclimatisation period of two weeks or so, well before the event, with subsequent shorter exposures nearer the contest. If this is not practicable, attempts should be made at some degree of heat acclimatisation before the athlete leaves for the host country. This may be achieved by "pre-acclimatisation".

On first exposure to a hot climate, athletes should be encouraged to drink copiously to maintain a pale straw-coloured rather than dark urine. They should drink much more fluid than they think they need, since thirst is often a very poor indicator of real need. On arrival in the hot country, athletes should be strongly discouraged from sunbathing as this itself does not help acclimatisation except as a means of acquiring a suntan, which eventually protects the skin from damage via solar radiation. This long-term process is not beneficial in the short-term, but negative effects of sunburn include discomfort and a decline in performance. Use of sunscreen is recommended for those likely to be exposed to the risk of sunburn.

Initially, training should be undertaken in the cooler parts of the day for an adequate workload to be achieved and adequate fluid must be taken regularly. Arrangements should be made to sleep in an air-conditioned environment, but, to acclimatise adequately, parts of the day should be spent exposed to the ambient temperature rather than in air-conditioned rooms. Although sweating increases with acclimatisation, salt tablets are not necessary provided adequate amounts of salt are taken with normal food.

In the acclimatisation period, the athlete should regularly monitor body weight and try to compensate for weight loss with adequate fluid intake. Alcohol is inappropriate for rehydration purposes, since it is a diuretic that increases urine output. Athletes can check that the volume of urine is as large as usual and its colour is normal. Groups using warm weather training camps should have urine osmolality (or conductance) monitored regularly to gauge hydration status.

The thermal strain on the individual depends on the relative exercise intensity (% VO_2max) rather than the absolute workload. The higher the maximal aerobic power (VO_2max) and cardiac output, the lower the thermal strain on the athlete. Well trained individuals have a highly developed cardiovascular system to cope with the dual roles of thermoregulation and oxygen delivery. Highly trained individuals also acclimatise more quickly than those who are unfit. Training improves exercise tolerance in the heat, but does not eliminate the necessity for heat acclimatisation.

Heat injury

Hyperthermia (overheating) and loss of body water (hypohydration) lead to abnormalities referred to as heat injury. Progressively, these may be manifest as muscle cramps, heat exhaustion, and heat stroke. They are observed more frequently in individual events, such as distance running and cycling, than in field games.

Heat cramps are associated with loss of body fluid, particularly when competing in intense heat. Although the body loses electrolytes in sweat, such losses cannot adequately account for cramps occurring. Cramps generally coincide with low energy stores as well as dehydration. The muscles employed in the exercise are usually affected, especially the leg (upper or lower) and abdominal muscles. Cramps can be stopped by stretching the involved muscle; sometimes massage is effective.

Heat exhaustion is characterised by a core temperature of about 40°C. There is a feeling of extreme tiredness, dizziness,

Main effects of heat acclimatisation
• Blood volume ↑
• Sweat rate ↑
onset at a lower core temperature
greater distribution over body surface
• Sodium and chloride content of sweat and urine ↓
• Perception of effort ↓
• Glycogen utilisation ↓

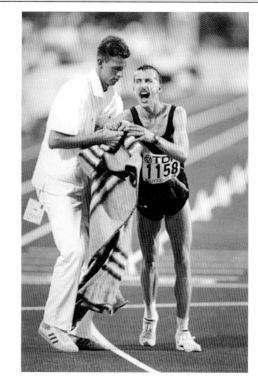

Figure 14.4

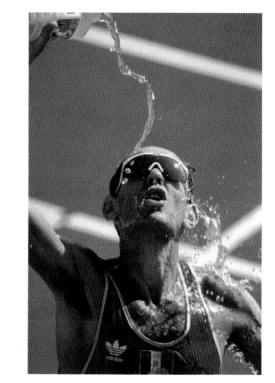

Figure 14.5

breathlessness, and tachycardia (increased heart rate). The symptoms may coincide with reduced sweat loss, but usually arise because the skin blood vessels are so dilated that blood flow to vital organs is reduced.

Heat stroke is a true medical emergency. It is characterised by core temperatures of 41°C or higher. Hypohydration—due to loss of body water in sweat and associated with a high core temperature—can threaten life. Heat stroke is characterised by cessation of sweating, total confusion, or unconsciousness. Treatment is urgently needed to reduce body temperature. There may also be circulatory instability and loss of vasomotor tone as the regulation of blood pressure fails.

All racial groups are vulnerable to heat stress. West African athletes, for example, lose their tolerance to heat stress during the rainy season. In hot conditions, the rise in temperature can be the factor that limits performance.

Monitoring environmental temperature

In order to evaluate the environmental heat load on the athlete, an integrated assessment is required. Many equations have been devised for this purpose, the most widely held being the WBGT Index (wet, bulb, and globe temperature). The weightings underline the importance of the relative humidity. In the USA, guidelines for distance running indicate that races longer than 16 km (10 miles) should be abandoned when the WBGT index exceeds 28°C. Many sports events are held in more extreme conditions, although the tendency is to organise competitive marathons during the morning, when the environmental stress is more tolerable.

The WBGT Index

WBGT = 0.7 WBT + 0.2 GBT + 0.1 DBT	
Where	WB represents wet bulb
	G indicates globe
	DB represents dry bulb
	T indicates temperature

Heat disorders

Heat cramps

- Muscle spasms (usually in the unacclimatised)

Heat syncope

- General weakness and fatigue; brief loss of consciousness

Heat exhaustion

- Dizzy; tired; breathless; reduced sweat loss
- Reduced blood flow to vital organs
- Loss of coordination
- Rise in heart rate; vasodilation

Heat stroke

- Confused and irrational
- Skin and core temperature high; dry skin
- Pale blue colour
- May hallucinate
- May stop sweating
- Medical emergency

Individuals particularly at risk of heat stress

- Previous sufferers of heat illness
- Unacclimatised individuals
- Untrained individuals
- Dehydrated individuals
- Individuals with a high percent body fat
- Persons with viral illness
- Individuals on medication, for example diuretics; antihistamines

15 Temperature and performance: cold

Thomas Reilly

Competing in cold

Besides the so-called winter sports, many games are often played in near freezing conditions. Furthermore, recreational activities, such as hill walking, may entail exposure to low environmental temperatures and there is a risk of cold water immersion with boating accidents. Core and muscle temperatures may fall and exercise performance is increasingly affected; consciousness is impaired as core temperature drops to its lower safe limit of 35°C. Hypothermia is life-threatening and the body's heat gain mechanisms are designed to arrest the body temperature decline.

With the fall in limb temperature arising from cutaneous vasoconstriction, motor performance declines. Muscle power output is reduced by 5% for every 1°C fall in muscle temperature below normal. Along with the drop in muscular strength and power output as the temperature in the muscle falls, conduction velocity of nerve impulses to the muscles is slowed. Sensitivity of muscle spindles also declines and manual dexterity is impaired. Limb temperatures can be preserved by wearing appropriate gloves.

The thermoregulatory responses to cold are initiated by the "heat gain centre" in the posterior hypothalamus. A generalised peripheral vasoconstriction of the cutaneous circulation, mediated by the sympathetic nervous system, displaces blood from shell to core in response to cold. The decrease in peripheral blood flow reduces heat loss to the environment, but the changes in blood flow are not uniform throughout the body. Flow to the fingers may decline by a factor of 40 compared with normal whereas, with no vasoconstricor fibres to the scalp, blood flow to the head remains unaltered. Consequently, heat loss through the head contributes to hypothermia in cold conditions and covering the head is some protection.

Shivering is a response of the body's autonomic nervous system to falling core temperature. It constitutes involuntary activity of skeletal muscles to generate metabolic heat. Shivering tends to be intermittent and persists during exercise if the intensity is insufficient to maintain core temperature. It may be evident during stoppages in activity.

Early symptoms of hypothermia include shivering, fatigue, loss of strength and coordination, and an inability to sustain work-rate. Diuresis accompanies a prolonged exposure to cold. Once fatigue develops, shivering may decrease and the condition worsens. Later symptoms include collapse, stupor, and loss of consciousness. Particularly vulnerable are individuals who are unable to sustain a work-rate to keep themselves warm in extreme cold.

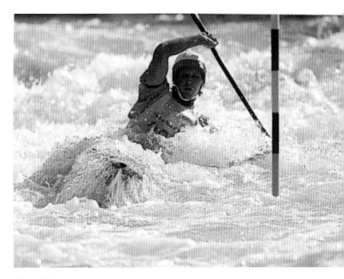

Figure 15.1

Selected effects of cold on human performance
- Peripheral vasoconstriction ↑
- Metabolism ↑
- Shivering (periodic)
- Muscle spindle sensitivity ↓
- Nerve conduction velocity—delayed
- Manual dexterity ↓
- Muscle strength/power ↓
- Accidents ↑

Coping with cold conditions

Cold is less problematic than heat since the body may be protected against exposure to the ambient environment. The microclimate surrounding the skin is critical; it may be maintained by appropriate choice of clothing. Behaviourally, individuals might respond to cold by maintaining a high work-rate. Alternatively, games players may be spared exposure to cold by training in available indoor facilities.

Clothing made of natural fibre (cotton or wool) is preferable to synthetic material in cold and in cold-wet conditions. The clothing should allow sweat produced during exercise in these conditions to flow through the garment. The best material will allow sweat to flow out through the cells of the garment while preventing water droplets from penetrating the clothing from the outside. If the fabric becomes saturated with water or sweat, it loses its insulation and in cold-wet conditions body temperature may quickly drop.

Athletes training in the cold should keep the trunk area of the body well insulated. Warm undergarments may be worn beneath a full tracksuit. Dressing in layers is advised; outer layers can be discarded as body temperature rises and if the ambient temperature rises.

When layers of clothing are worn, the outer layer should be capable of resisting both wind and rain. The inner layer should provide insulation and also wick moisture from the skin to promote heat loss by evaporation. Polypropylene and cotton fishnet thermal underwear, having good insulation and wicking properties, is suitable to wear next to the skin.

Immediately prior to competing in the cold, games players should stay warm. A thorough warm-up (performed indoors if possible) is recommended. Cold increases the risk of muscle injury in sports involving anaerobic efforts; warm-up exercises afford some protection against injury. Competitors may need to wear more clothing than they normally do during matches.

Water immersion

Water has a 25-fold greater heat conduction capacity than air and a specific heat 4000 times greater, and therefore heat is readily exchanged with the environment when the human body is immersed. The preferred water temperature for inactive individuals is 32–33°C, for those learning to swim it is about 30°C, for active swimmers 27°C, and for competitive swimmers 25°C. Nevertheless, it is usual to keep the water temperature in public pools at 30°C. High humidity in swimming pools protects the swimmers against heat loss when out of the water, but is not optimal for the comfort of spectators. Air temperature in the region 28–30°C accentuates this.

The greater the swimming intensity, the lower is the water temperature for greatest efficiency. This relationship is influenc- ed by the physique and body composition of the swimmer. Lean swimmers are unable to maintain VO_2max at a water temperature of 26°C; fatter subjects show a similar failure at 18°C. The muscle mass complements the subcutaneous adipose tissue layers in insulating the body and prolongs exposure time in accidental immersion. The adipose tissue is relatively under- perfused; fat has a thermal conductivity half that of skeletal muscle and one third that of blood, so the thickness of the subcutaneous layer determines the heat flow from the body to the water.

Muscle function is adversely influenced by cold water immersion, grip strength in water as low as 2°C falling

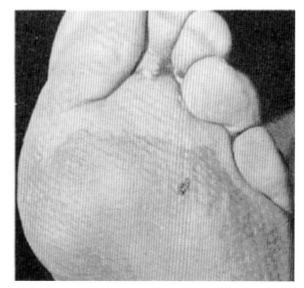

Figure 15.2 Cold rigid foot without sensation or digital motion. Note marks of sock texture. Extensive clear blisters developed, which became black when dry but finally sloughed off leaving normal function and anatomy. (Blood filled blisters, however, are a bad sign)

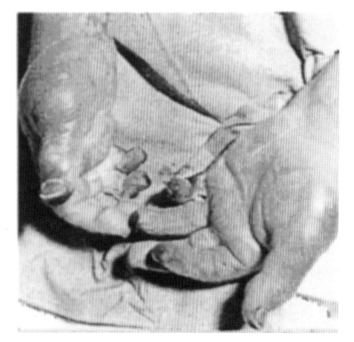

Figure 15.3 Hands less than 24 hours after frostbite thawed by using excess heat (boiling water in this case). Hands are cyanotic, painful, and foul smelling, and there are no blebs. Resulted in spontaneous amputation at the metacarpophalangeal junction at six weeks

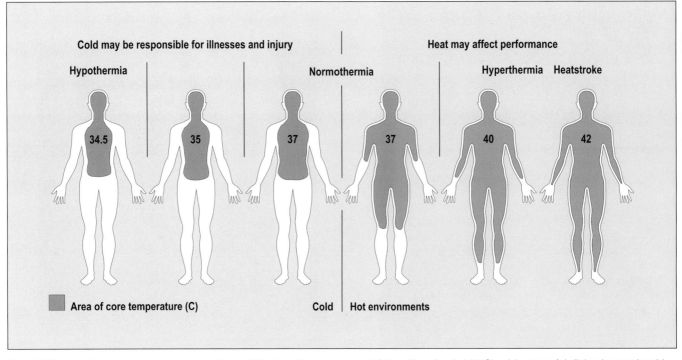

Figure 15.4 Rough relation of core temperatures and shell sizes. (Note the arbitrary temperature definition of hypothermia (<35°C) and the range of shell sizes in normothermia)

quickly to half the normal value. Muscle fatigue curves are detrimentally affected by an 8 minute immersion at 10°C but complete recovery occurs within 40 minutes. As muscle temperature falls below 27°C, muscle spindles respond to only 50% of normal to a standard stimulus, thereby affecting coordination. The fall in finger temperature will be even more pronounced, severely impairing manual dexterity.

Cold pathologies

Frostbite

Frostbite refers to a destruction of superficial tissues that can occur when the temperature in the fingers or toes falls below freezing and at -1°C ice crystals are formed in those tissues. The results can be a gangrenous extremity, often experienced by mountaineers in icy conditions when their gloves or boots fail to provide adequate thermal insulation. Recent clinical experience is that amputation of damaged tissue is not a necessary consequence of frostbite and prognosis tends to be more optimistic than thought in previous decades.

A fall in the body's core temperature is a more serious consequence. The cold stress is manifested progressively by an enlargement of the area of the shell, while the area of the core becomes smaller until its temperature ultimately begins to fall dangerously low. A core temperature of 34.5°C is usually taken as indicative of grave hypothermic risk, although there is no absolute consensus of a critical end point; the exact value of hypothalamic temperature for fatality is subject to controversy.

In cases of severe hypothermia, there is a risk of later circulatory, respiratory, and renal failure. The immediate aim must be to get the individual to shelter, provide hot fluid and extra clothing, and consider means of evacuation to hospital.

Adaptation to cold

Acclimatisation to cold is much less pronounced than to heat; behavioural and proper clothing strategies can safeguard

Cold pathologies
- Cold exhaustion
  - lowered body temperature
  - hypoglycaemia
  - cerebral function
  - motor coordination
  - confusion
  - accidents
- Frostbite
  - skin temperature–freezing point
  - intense local vasoconstriction
  - contact with cold material

individuals in cold environments. Physiological adaptations can occur, starting at the first experience of cold conditions.

Thyroxine increases metabolic rate within 5–6 hours of cold exposure. The elevated thyroxine output persists throughout the sojourn. Adrenaline and adrenocorticoid hormones contribute to the increase in metabolic rate. A thermogenic reaction to the secretion of noradrenaline develops from prolonged exposure, but the main response of habituated individuals is peripheral vasoconstriction in the cold.

Monitoring environmental cold stress

On the mountainside, the air velocity may be the most influential variable in cooling the body and measuring the ambient temperature, only it would greatly underestimate the prevailing risk. The "wind chill index" has provided skiers, mountaineers and hill walkers with a useful warning system for over half a century. The method entails comparing different combinations of temperature and wind speed. Calculated values correspond to a caloric scale for rate of heat loss relative to body surface area. The figures are converted to a sensation scale ranging from hot (about 80) through cool (400) to bitterly cold (1200) and up to a value where exposed flesh freezes within 60 seconds. Wet conditions can exacerbate cold stress, especially if the clothing worn loses its insulation.

Preparing for cold conditions

It is important to plan in detail for expeditions in cold conditions. For short-term exposures, weather forecasts are helpful. As the weather conditions can change quite quickly, for example, on the sea or mountainside, the worst of possible conditions should be catered for. Expedition leaders have particular responsibilities for calculating necessary provisions, clothing, and loads to be transported or carried. In inclement weather, when conditions deteriorate, original plans need to be modified to reduce risks of cold exposure and hypothermia.

Acknowledgements

The photographs are reproduced with permission of Allsport and Dr William J Mills Jnr, Anchorage, Alaska.

Wind chill formula for calculating heat loss	
$K_0 = (\sqrt{100V} + 10.5 - V)(33 - T)$	
Where	K_0 = heat loss in kcal/h
	V = wind velocity in m/s
	T = environmental temperature in °C
	10.5 = a constant
	33 = assumed normal skin temperature in °C

16 Groin pain

Vijay Kurup, Greg McLatchie, O J A Gilmore

Groin pain is a common problem among sportspeople. About five percent of all sports injuries are groin related. Accurate diagnosis is often difficult because many pathological processes in and around the groin area can precipitate similar types of pain. These can be vague and diffuse, or focal and well localised. If not treated the condition may become chronic and affect the sports career of the individual. Although many activities can cause groin injuries most are encountered in soccer, rugby, athletics, skating, cricket, running, horse riding, and general fitness training.

Aetiological factors

Hernia

Sportsmen complaining of pain in the groin could have a hernia. An indirect inguinal hernia that becomes irreducible can produce groin pain. Patients with a direct inguinal hernia notice discomfort, particularly with prolonged standing or slow walking as opposed to during more energetic sporting activities. Occasionally, a patient will have a femoral hernia and, rarely, an obturator hernia. Patients with an inguinal hernia have a palpable lump with a cough impulse on standing, while femoral hernias are irreducible, presenting as a lump below and lateral to the pubic tubercle. Patients with a symptomatic hernia require surgical repair.

Musculotendinous injuries

Soft tissue injuries account for the majority of groin symptoms in sports people. Tendon injuries are often "overuse" injuries. Tendinitis is the result of an injury or degeneration of the tendon resulting in an inflammatory reaction in the surrounding para-tenon. Onset of the pain can be acute, sub-acute, or chronic (2 weeks, 2–6 weeks, or >6 weeks). In addition to tendinitis, rupture of the tendons is also not uncommon in sportspeople. Rupture can be either partial or complete.

Adductor longus strain

This is a common occurrence and is often a result of external rotation and abduction injuries. High kicks and sliding tackles in soccer, repetitive abduction in skating, and horse riding predisposes to adductor longus injuries. Skiing only causes adductor strains if there is a fall. People who ski properly keep their legs together and, therefore, do not suffer abduction injuries. Onset of pain may follow a single incident or will be insidious in origin. Pain in the groin is located in the adductor insertion region and exacerbated by wide separation of the legs. Tenderness around the origin of adductor longus in the pubic bone is characteristic. The symptoms are reproduced by resisted adduction.

> **Differential diagnosis**
>
> - Hernia
> - Musculotendinous injuries
>   - adductor tendinitis/rupture
>   - rectus femoris strain
>   - rectus abdominis strain
>   - iliopsoas strain
>   - enthesopathy—inguinal ligament
>   - osteitis symphysis pubis
>   - pubic instability
>   - bursitis
>   - groin disruption
> - Hip and spinal pathology
> - Nerve entrapments
> - Fractures
> - Systemic causes
>   - gastrointestinal
>   - urological
>   - gynaecological
> - Testicular

Rectus abdominis strain

Sporting events involving repetitive flexion movements at the groin, such as sit-ups and leg raises, can lead to rectus abdominis strain. Pain and tenderness is noted over the insertion of the muscle into the pubic bone. Symptoms are exacerbated by hip flexion against resistance.

Iliopsoas strain

This can occur when the hip is actively flexed, or when the hip is forcefully flexed against resistance. Pain and tenderness is vague and diffuse and often experienced deep in the groin at the site of insertion on the lesser trochanter. Repeated sit-ups and rowing machine exercises are known to cause iliopsoas strain. Hip flexion against resistance may reproduce the symptoms.

Rectus femoris strain

The rectus femoris can be damaged at its origin on the upper half of the anterior inferior iliac spine. These injuries are often seen in association with sprint starts in runners and kicking episodes in soccer players. Pain and tenderness is noted over the muscle origin and exacerbated by resisted hip flexion.

Inguinal ligament

Enthesopathy or inflammation at the insertion of inguinal ligament in the pubic bone can also lead to chronic groin pain. Usually, the pain is diffuse and ill localised.

Osteitis pubis

This condition is related to instability and inflammation of the pubic symphysis. It is seen in adolescents and young adults who undertake vigorous training. Pain and tenderness is experienced over the pubic symphysis or along the pubic ramus.

Bursitis

There are eight bursae around the hip joint in relation to the attachment of deep tendons. They can undergo inflammatory changes and produce chronic groin pain. Trochanteric bursae and the bursae around the insertion of iliopsoas are the ones most often involved. These are difficult to diagnose and usually associated with muscular damage.

Groin disruption (Gilmore's Groin)

Groin disruption may be defined as a condition involving musculotendinous injuries of the groin area leading to chronic pain in sportspeople. The pain can be so disabling that at times the relevant sporting activity will have to be discontinued. It is also known as "Gilmore's Groin" or "Sports Hernia". The pathologies described in groin disruption include:

- Torn external oblique aponeurosis
- Torn conjoined tendon
- A dilated superficial inguinal ring
- A dehiscence between inguinal ligament and conjoined tendon
- The absence of a hernia sac.

Groin disruption is usually an "overuse" injury. Repeated stretching of the posterior wall in the inguinal canal over a long period of time results in widening of the external ring due to tearing of the external oblique aponeurosis. The conjoined tendon is formed by the union of the internal oblique and transversus abdominis muscle as a tendinous insertion at the pubic crease extending along the pectineal line. A torn conjoined tendon can be considered to be the same as a posterior wall defect at the medial margin of the inguinal canal region. Although there is musculotendinous disruption, a proper hernial sac is not described as part of Gilmore's Groin nor is it necessary that all these pathologies should occur at the same time.

In studies on soccer players, we have shown the underlying problem in groin disruption is muscle imbalance and overuse. The strong hip flexors that are used to kick the ball tilt the pelvis forward; the forward pelvis stretches the abdominal muscles, which become weak and fail to stabilise the pelvis. Excessive physical activity results in tears of the groin muscles, tendons, and ligaments and thus groin disruption. Because of the underlying muscle imbalance, these patients may also have hamstring problems (recurrent tears) and back problems (often lordosis).

Degenerative changes of hip and spine

In some cases, osteoarthritis affecting the lumbosacral spine and hip joint can be responsible for chronic pain in the groin area. Intervertebral disc prolapse irritating the spinal nerve roots can also lead to intractable groin pain.

Nerve entrapment

The ilioinguinal, iliohypogastric, genitofemoral, obturator and lateral cutaneous nerve of the thigh can become involved in

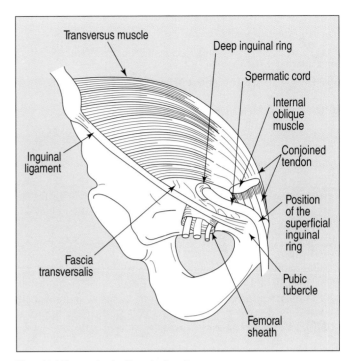

Figure 16.1 The area involved in groin disruption

entrapment syndromes, which may, in turn, cause groin pain. There is often a history of previous surgery, such as appendicectomy, hernia repair or a Pfanneustiel incision. These incisions may be associated with nerve injury, subsequent entrapment, or neuroma formation. A local anaesthetic injection that relieves the pain may be used as a diagnostic test. In some patients exploration of the area with excision of the involved nerve may also be necessary to establish a cure.

In other patients, where there is no history of previous surgery, high entrapment in the fascia lata is a possible cause of groin pain relieved by surgical release. Gymnasts, in particular, can develop meralgia paraesthetica due to entrapment of, or trauma to, the lateral cutaneous nerve of the thigh when practising on asymmetric bars. A period of four to six weeks of an altered training programme usually allows the condition to settle.

Fractures

Rigorous sporting activities can lead to both stress and avulsion fractures. Fractures involving the pelvis and neck of the femur can lead to chronic or acute groin pain. Stress fractures are increasingly seen in long distance runners and joggers, especially females. In the pelvis, these fractures are almost invariably of the inferior pubic ramus close to the symphysis. Pain may be experienced in the groin, buttock, or thigh during or after training. Movements of the hip, particularly external rotation and abduction, are limited due to pain.

Stress fractures of the femoral neck are commonly encountered in long distance runners, hurdlers, skiers, and football players. The plain X-ray may be negative in the initial weeks. Pain is experienced in the groin extending to the anterior thigh and sometimes to the knee. Compression fractures of the femoral neck are not uncommon. These are usually located at the medial margin of the cortex of the femoral neck and are frequently seen in younger athletes.

Slipped upper femoral epiphysis

This should be considered in adolescents as an uncommon cause of groin pain.

Systemic causes

Lower gastrointestinal diseases
Diverticular disease, inflammatory bowel disease, appendicitis, mesenteric lymphadenitis and, occasionally, bowel malignancies can give rise to groin pain.

Urological causes
Ureteric calculi, urinary tract infections, and prostatitis should be considered in the differential diagnosis and excluded.

Gynaecological causes
Chronic groin pain in women may be caused by pelvic inflammatory disease, endometriosis, or disease of the uterus, tubes, or ovaries. Ultrasound scanning of the pelvic contents and referral to a gynaecologist is appropriate.

Testicular causes
Epididymo-orchitis, varicocoeles, trauma and, occasionally, tumours can all cause groin pain. The history and examination will confirm a testicular cause. Ultrasound screening of the testes is useful for detecting small tumours, the most common form of malignancy in young men.

Investigations

Plain films
Plain films of the pelvis, hip joints, and lumbosacral spine will confirm the presence of fracture, avulsion, ectopic calcification, or degenerative change. In osteitis pubis, there is widening and fragmentation or sclerotic changes of the pubic symphysis. Stork or flamingo views taken with the patient standing on one leg then the other can demonstrate pelvic instability. If there is more than 4 mm displacement, this may be significant and orthopaedic advice should be sought.

Ultrasound scan
This can detect haematoma, cysts, hernia, varicocoele, hydrocoele, and also testicular tumours.

Bone scanning
Radioisotope (Tech- 99) bone scanning can identify osteitis pubis, avulsion and stress fractures as well as early degenerative changes affecting the spine and other joints that may not be seen clearly on plain X-rays.

Herniography
In this invasive investigation, contrast is introduced into the peritoneal cavity through a subumbilical puncture wound. The patient is then screened radiologically for evidence of a hernia sac. The procedure is useful in obscure or undetected hernias, but the success rate depends on the expertise of the radiologist. However, it is not diagnostic in groin disruption.

Magnetic resonance imaging (MRI)
MRI scans of the pelvis and the soft tissues of the groin are assuming an increasingly important role in the evaluation of groin injuries. MRI scans can identify muscle and tendon injuries, bone and joint diseases, and can give clues to groin disruption. Certain aspects of groin disruption, such as widening of the external ring and inguinal canal and disruption of the external oblique, can be identified by an experienced radiologist.

Investigations
- Plain X-ray
  - hip and pelvis
  - stork views
- Bone scan
- Ultrasound scan
  - groin and testes
- Herniography
- MRI scan

Appropriate investigations to exclude systemic pathology have to be considered. These include IVU, cystoscopy, colonoscopy, CT scanning, and MRI scanning of the relevant areas.

Treatment

Musculotendinous injuries
'Groin strain' implies injury to any of the following muscles; the sartorius, any or all of the adductors (rider's strain), the long head of rectus femoris, the iliopsoas, and any of the abdominal muscles. A tear of the adductor muscles usually occurs around the musculotendinous junction about 5 cm from the pubis or, less commonly, at the tendo-osseous junction producing pain around the pubic tubercle or superior ramus.

Groin injuries can present acutely as a result of overstretching, twisting or lunging. The diagnosis is made by the presence of local tenderness with pain on resisted contraction of isolated muscles. Chronic injuries are more difficult to evaluate and may involve more than one pathological process. Most groin problems present acutely.

During the acute phase the standard principles of soft tissue injury management should be followed for the first 48–72 hours. These include "functional" rather than complete rest if possible. Any activity that stresses the injured area should be avoided and crutches can be used in severe cases to limit use of the injured part. Cooling of the injury with ice or cold water reduces hypoxic tissue damage and provides local analgesia. Ice packs should be applied for 15–20 minutes every two hours for the first two days. If possible, compression should also be applied and the injured area elevated. Analgesics or anti-inflammatory drugs are effective during the first 72 hours after injury.

Gentle movements within the limits of pain can begin following the acute phase, the aim being to facilitate repair of the soft tissue. This phase of healing lasts between 72 hours to six weeks. Passive and active stretching should be encouraged to limit muscle tightness that can delay return to sport. This rehabilitation should begin as soon as the reduction in pain allows.

At this stage, physiotherapeutic modalities may include massage, ultrasound, and electrical muscle stimulation with clear instructions to the patient regarding limitation of activity. When the repair phase is complete, the intensity of exercise can be safely increased to permit tissue remodelling, a return to general fitness and psychological well-being. Patients should be forewarned that the injury may take between four to eight weeks to heal.

Surgery is indicated for the reattachment of significant avulsion injuries or repair of ruptured tendons or muscle tears.

Osteitis pubis is best managed by rest, the symptoms settling in several weeks or months. If there is significant pelvic instability on weight bearing (>4 mm shift), plating or bone grafting may be considered.

Symptomatic hernias should be surgically repaired. Bassini, Shouldice, Mesh, or Laparoscopic repair may be chosen according to individual preference. However, the aim should be to achieve a tensionless repair.

Groin disruption

Conservative treatment is often unsuccessful and surgical intervention gives good results. Exploration of the groin is performed and individual pathologies are identified and rectified: repair of external oblique aponeurosis and reconstitution of the superficial inguinal ring, repair of the conjoint tendon, plication of the transversalis fascia and Nylon® darn repair of the posterior wall of the inguinal canal approximating conjoint tendon and inguinal ligament. A strict rehabilitation programme under the supervision of a physiotherapist must be followed postoperatively.

Skeletal injuries

These require treatment by orthopaedic surgeons. Fractures can be treated conservatively if there is no significant distraction between bone ends. Sometimes internal fixation will be required followed by a rehabilitation programme.

Summary

Groin pain is a significant symptom in sportsmen and women which frequently causes inability to participate and can lead to retirement from sport. Financially, there is likely to be loss of earnings for both the professional sportsplayer and the manual worker due to the restriction of activity that the condition imposes. The psychological impact of being unable to play sport can also lead to depression especially if financial loss results from the injury. The incidence is increasing because fewer players now take breaks between seasons. However, doctors and physiotherapists are becoming increasingly aware of the significance and nature of groin injuries and of the need to identify those patients (with groin disruption) who will respond well to surgical repair. Reports from different centres around the world have indicated that, with careful evaluation, surgical treatment where required and an appropriate rehabilitation programme, most sports players with different types of groin injury can successfully return to their previous level of activity.

References

Gilmore OJA (1998) Groin pain in the soccer athlete: fact, fiction and treatment. *Clin Sports Med* **17**(4): 787–93

Gilmore OJA. (1999) Groin disruption in sportsmen. In: Kurzer M, Kark A, Wantz G, eds. *Surgical Management of Abdominal Wall Hernias*. Martin Dunitz, London: 151–7

Renstrom P (1992) Tendon and muscle injuries in the groin area. *Clin Sports Med* **11**(4): 815–31

Urquhart DS, Packer GT, McLatchie GR (1996) Return to sport and patient satisfaction levels after surgical treatment for groin disruption. *Sports Exer Inj* **2**(37): 42

Groin disruption rehabilitation programme

Week 1	First day after operation: essential to stand upright and walk for 20 minutes Thereafter, walk gently 4 times a day. Gentle stretching exercises given by physiotherapists to be followed
Week 2	Jogging and gentle running in straight lines Gentle sit-ups with knees bent Adductor exercises Step-ups
Week 3	Increase speed to sprinting Increase sit-ups and adductor exercises Cycling Swimming (crawl)
Week 4	Sprint Twist and turn Kick Play

17 Team medical care

Malcolm W Brown

Medical care for a sports team should be a continuous process. Care at and around the time of the sporting contest is the most visible aspect of the medical team's responsibility. Ideally, this should follow on seamlessly from out-of-competition support during the rest of the year. The size and shape of the medical team will inevitably vary from sport to sport. It will reflect the varied medical requirements of different types of athletes, but will also be influenced by the financial resources available. As a result, what is possible for a large premier division soccer club will require drastic tailoring to suit a small amateur team. The descriptions in this chapter will reflect the current experience in British athletics (track and field) and falls somewhere between the two extremes.

Structure of the medical team

The medical support team, although usually led by a doctor, will only function optimally if it is truly multi-professional and non-hierarchical. Other members of the team will include physiotherapists, masseurs, podiatrists, sports dieticians and psychologists. Sports scientists, such as exercise physiologists and biomechanical experts, may either be part of the medical team, or more closely aligned with the coaching side of the sport. In the latter case, effective dialogue between the two groups is essential. It may at times be helpful to convene 'case conferences' where each member of the team provides input from their own professional perspective. Feedback can then be given to the athlete (and ideally his/her coach).

Out-of-competition support

The regular multi-professional support team may be able to deal with all the primary care for medical problems that arise throughout the season. This is more likely when teams are small and when regular squad sessions are held, or where the geographic distribution of players and support staff is favourable. For larger teams spread around the country, the medical team may principally act as coordinators of medical care, facilitating access to specialists conveniently located for the athlete.

Organisation of an effective support system will depend on a commonsense approach to matching available resources with access to specialist services. Rapid access to specialist advice and treatment should be made a priority. This may involve subscribing to a medical insurance scheme. Provision for physiotherapy support at regular intervals throughout the year may have to be developed separately, if not allowed for under the terms of the insurance scheme. If possible, this arrangement should allow proactive treatment of imbalances and potential problems rather than being totally reactive in response to injuries.

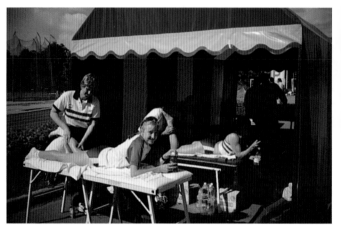

Figure 17.1

Medical team
- Doctor
- Physiotherapists
- Masseurs
- Podiatrist
- Sports dietician
- Psychologist

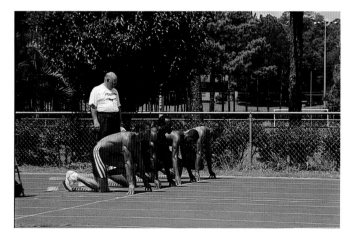

Figure 17.2

Screening sessions

Routine screening sessions for each athlete can be valuable, particularly if these can be repeated at regular intervals. Screening, in this sense, should adhere to standard principles and should, therefore, concentrate on the detection of common and remediable problems using appropriately sensitive tests. This may not necessarily involve large batteries of blood tests on essentially healthy individuals. The approach in athletics is that, during a screening session, each athlete rotates through various stations seeing the physiotherapist, doctor, podiatrist, sports dietician, and psychologist in turn. The professional involved may be able to deal with a particular problem there and then, but often identifying the need for further investigation or planned treatment will be more appropriate.

Education

Any contact with the athlete can be regarded as a potential educational opportunity. This may be constructed formally as a lecture to a group on a particular topic. Opportunities for education may occur during the screening sessions and also during more casual conversations with team members, such as during mealtimes or while travelling to the competition venue. The key to effective education is presenting the right message at the right time, i.e. when the athlete is in receptive mode. The doctor or therapist transmitting the message must first of all have established their credentials and be considered approachable and knowledgeable by the athlete. Bear in mind that athletes will often approach another athlete of stature for information on a particular subject and it may, at times, be necessary to contradict previously given advice of this type.

Competition support

Medical team

The medical team selected for competition support will ideally be the same individuals who are involved in caring for the athletes between competitions. This may not always be possible, or practical, and particular attention must be paid to effective communication between the various professionals involved before and after the competition in question. In theory, the treatments required during competition should only involve maintenance physiotherapy and massage with first aid and continuing treatment for any new problems arising. However, due to the pressures involved, it is not uncommon for the elite athlete to arrive at the venue a few days before the championship, requiring treatment for a significant problem that threatens to prevent his/her participation.

Preparation for travel and competition

Prior to travelling to the competition, advice should be given by the team doctor on necessary vaccinations and the environmental hazards of the particular venue. These may include high altitude, heat and humidity, allergens, and infective hazards. For long journeys, particularly for inexperienced teams, advice on coping with long flights and changes in time zones might be necessary. Jet lag will significantly impair performance and time must be allowed for re-setting the body clock and acclimatisation to difficult environmental conditions.

Equipment

At some competition venues, there may be a high level of support provided by the local organisers. At the Olympic Games, it is normal for a "polyclinic" to be set up within the Olympic Village and this will provide facilities equivalent to a hospital outpatient

> **Out-of-competition support**
> - Coordinate medical care throughout season
> - Facilitate access to specialists
> - Provide primary care if practical
> - May require private medical insurance
> - Able to access all members of the medical team
> - Regular screening allows proactive approach
> - Make the most of educational opportunities

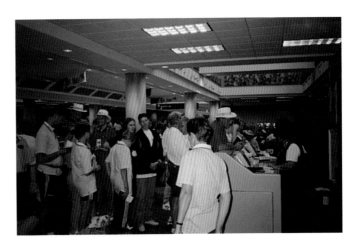

Figure 17.3

department with access to a pharmacy, specialist laboratory investigations, and radiological investigations, including MRI or CT. Access is also provided to various specialists, such as orthopaedic surgeons, general physicians, ophthalmologists, and dentists.

At most smaller competitions, it is usually best if the medical team can be self-sufficient and bring along any equipment that may be required. This will usually include portable physiotherapy tables and any electrical equipment that might be used.

Medical bag

The contents of the team doctor's bag will evolve over time, with new additions being made on each subsequent trip as, inevitably, there will be something that you wish you had included. This could lead to transporting a mini-pharmacy from country to country. A sensible compromise would be to carry small quantities of drugs to cover the most common minor ailments likely to afflict a team of young, healthy individuals. It is important to be aware of the restrictions placed on prescribing by the anti-doping regulations and it seems sensible to carry only medicines that would be allowed under the regulations of the particular sport. This approach can, however, lead to problems if it is ever necessary to administer strong analgesics following a particularly painful injury.

It is useful to carry an inventory of all drugs contained in the medical bag and this can be presented if any enquiries are made when negotiating customs.

Venue support and back-up

The medical team has ultimate responsibility for the care given to their athletes. On occasions, first-aid volunteers or a local medical team may provide immediate care if individual team doctors and physiotherapists are not allowed access to the competition arena. It is essential that the arrangements for clearance from the field of play are well established and team support staff must know where and when they will be able to access their athletes. Arrangements should be in place for transferring athletes to hospital should serious injury or illness occur that is beyond the scope of the support staff available at the competition venue.

Relationships with the coaches and managers

The relationship between an athlete and the team doctor is subject to the same rules of confidentiality as any doctor–patient relationship. However, when medical information may be relevant in terms of an athlete's future performance (especially when part of a team), the athlete should be encouraged to communicate with the team manager or coach, or ask the doctor to do so on his/her behalf.

The media

From time to time members of the media may ask the medical team for comment. Consent of the athlete concerned is essential and the medical team should also have established a strategy for dealing with such requests. It is not appropriate for individual members of the team to venture their opinions separately. The spokesperson for the team should either be the team leader (usually the doctor) or else all such communication should be via a press officer. When television is involved, a spot diagnosis may be sought in order to relay the information to the watching viewers. Under such occasions it is wise only to make very general comments and again only with the athlete's consent.

Doping issues

The team doctor will not normally be concerned with the actual carrying out of anti-doping tests. On the other hand, it is good

---

Competition support

- Ideally the same individuals as out-of-competition support
- Good communication regarding previous and on-going problems
- Provide advice on necessary vaccinations and environmental hazards
- Advise on strategy to minimise jet lag
- Medical team should aim for self-sufficiency
- Identify potential back-up arrangements for major problems

Medical bag

- Carry small supplies of drugs for all likely minor ailments
- Take larger supplies of certain drugs if particular problems are expected
- Have a generous supply of a suitable NSAID
- Avoid drugs on the 'banned list'
- Have available an inventory of the drugs carried when passing through customs

---

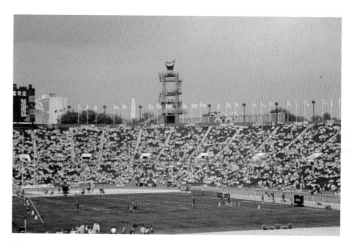

Figure 17.4

practice for the team doctor to accompany his/her athletes to Doping Control and observe the testing procedure to ensure there have been no irregularities and provide reassurance to the athlete being tested. It is useful to interview each athlete before the competition starts to ensure that no banned substances are inadvertently being taken and all necessary declarations have been made.

In the event of an adverse finding in a doping sample, the team doctor should offer general support and advice.

Further reading

Bird J, Verroken M (1998) *Competitors and Officials Guide to Drugs and Sport*. United Kingdom Sports Council, Walkden House, 10, Melton Street, London, UK

Dirix A, Knuttgen HG, Tittel K, eds (1988) *The Olympic Book of Sports Medicine*. Blackwell Scientific Publications, Oxford

Harries M, Williams C, Stanish WD, Micheli LJ, eds (1998) *Oxford Textbook of Sports Medicine*, 2nd edn. Oxford Medical Publications, Oxford

Manfredini R, Manfredini F, Fersini C, Conconi F (1998) Circadian rhythms, athletic performance and jet lag. *Br J Sports Med* **32**:101–6

Key points
- Team medical care should be a continuous process
- Includes out-of-competition support
- Non-hierarchical multi-professional teams work best
- Rapid access to specialist advice should be a priority
- Look to be proactive in injury prevention
- Regular screening may identify unsuspected problems
- Remember rules of confidentiality

18 Eye injuries in sport

Caroline J MacEwen

Introduction

Injuries to the eye that occur during sporting activities are a serious problem. Although the majority of such injuries are superficial, involving only the external eye or surrounding tissues, in approximately one third of cases there is damage to the intraocular structures with potentially sight-threatening consequences. Sport is currently responsible for between 25–40% of all eye injuries that are severe enough to require hospital admission. Most of these injuries are recognised as being entirely preventible.

Spectrum of injury

Superficial blunt trauma

The majority of all sporting eye injuries are caused by balls or collisions with other players and are, therefore, blunt in nature. The most common effect of such an injury is the periorbital contusion or 'black eye', which although not a serious injury, may cause tense eyelid swelling that prevents adequate examination of the underlying globe. As it is inadvisable to force the lids open, this may lead to a serious ocular injury being missed. Sub-conjunctival haemorrhage, easily recognised as a diffuse, uniform, bright red area covering some or all of the white of the eye, commonly occurs in association with a black-eye. The corneal epithelium is often disrupted or removed by a direct blow and this causes an acutely painful corneal abrasion (*Figure 18.1*).

Blow out fractures

Blow out fractures occur when the eye is struck with significant force and the intraorbital pressure rises abruptly so that the floor of the orbit 'blows out' into the maxillary antrum. It is accompanied by prolapse of the inferior contents orbital causing enophthalmos and double vision. Involvement of the infraorbital nerve results in anaesthesia of the second division of the fifth cranial nerve. X-rays of the orbit indicate the prolapse of tissue and opacity of the maxillary antrum due to blood. CT scans that give a clearer picture of the injury are required if surgery is considered necessary (*Figure 18.2*).

Intraocular blunt trauma

If the intraocular structures are damaged, the most frequent sign of severe blunt injury is the hyphaema, which is caused by bleeding into the anterior chamber (*Figure 18.3*). This is a common injury when the eye is struck by a squash ball or shuttlecock. The bleeding usually comes from a tear in the iris, but a hyphaema implies that significant intraocular trauma has occurred and urgent specialist attention is required.

A direct blow to the eye may cause a tear in the peripheral retina, predisposing to a retinal detachment. Similarly, damage to

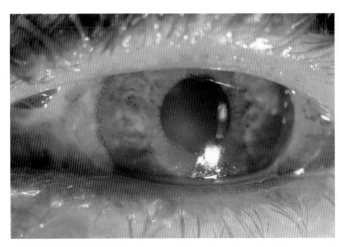

Figure 18.1 Corneal abrasion stained with fluorescein

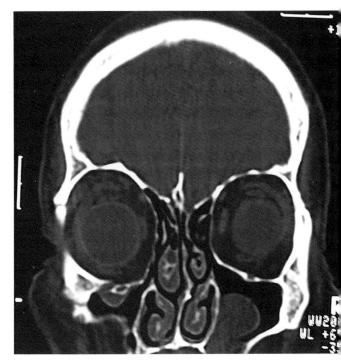

Figure 18.2 Scan of a blow out fracture of the orbital floor

retinal vessels may cause a vitreous haemorrhage. Commotio retina—traumatic oedema of the sensory retina (*Figure 18.4*)—can be extensive and, if the macular area is involved, carries a poor prognosis for visual recovery. Choroidal ruptures are common in the macular area, leading to considerable reduction in central vision (*Figure 18.5*). These posterior segment injuries usually occur after an injury with a heavy object, such as a football, and are also common in boxing. Severe blunt trauma results in rupture of the globe; the vision is dramatically reduced and there is severe subconjunctival bleeding and swelling.

Small foreign particles

Small pieces of foreign material, such as dust or grit, are often blown or flicked onto the eye during any outdoor activity. These little particles may remain on the cornea causing intense pain. In some instances, they settle under the upper lid as sub-tarsal foreign bodies and rub up and down scratching the front of the eye as it opens and closes.

Penetrating injuries

Penetrating injuries due to rackets, sticks, fingers, or fish hooks (*Figure 18.6*) entering the globe are fortunately rare. They should be suspected if the anterior chamber appears shallower on the injured side, or if the pupil is irregular, as the iris plugs the wound. The extent of injury depends on how far the object has entered the eye, but multiple intraocular structures are commonly affected, resulting in a poor visual outcome.

Burns

Skiers and climbers are susceptible to 'snow blindness' due to ultra-violet light burns causing corneal de-epithelialisation. Chemical burns are uncommon, but can occur in swimmers from excess chlorination of swimming pools and from particles of lime from the pitch markings that accidently enter the eye.

Assessment and first aid

The role of the attending doctor is to determine whether or not an eye injury is serious, to treat any minor injuries, and to sanction return to the field if considered appropriate. The eye should be examined in a systematic fashion, using a good light (*Figure 18.7*). Examination of the surface of the eye should be supplemented with a drop of fluorescein which will stain a corneal foreign body or abrasion as bright green, especially if viewed with a blue light (*Figure 18.1*). Corneal abrasions are extremely painful and it is unlikely that play will be resumed if one is sustained. Similarly, those with corneal foreign bodies will suspend play and it is inappropriate for these to be removed on the touch-line. In cases of superficial eye injury, a topical antibiotic eye ointment should be instilled to prevent secondary infection and a firm pad applied to keep the patient comfortable. If there is severe discomfort, the upper eyelid should be everted using a cotton bud and any foreign material sitting under the lid swept off. More diffuse conjunctival material, such as mud, is best removed by irrigating the eye with sterile saline. Contact lens wearers should have the lens found and removed from the affected eye.

Hyphaema may be evident as a level of blood within the anterior chamber (*Figure 18.3*), but, more commonly in the acute phase, as a cloudy anterior chamber with a hazy appearance to the iris. The pupils should be equal, round and react to light, and any irregularity should be considered a sign of intraocular damage.

Players with serious injuries should be transferred promptly to hospital for specialist attention. Any chemical irritant should be washed out of the eye as a matter of urgency before transfer and

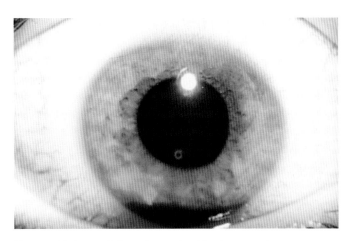
Figure 18.3 Hyphaema—indicates that a serious injury has occurred

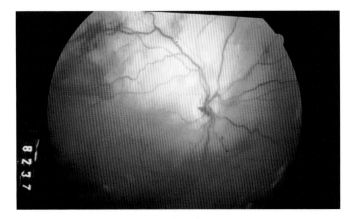
Figure 18.4 Area of commotio retina—pallor of the retina with associated haemorrhage

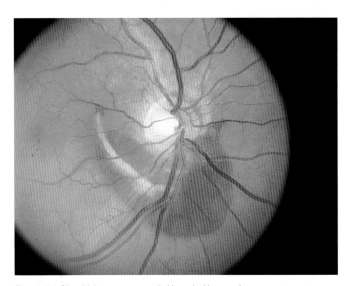
Figure 18.5 Choroidal rupture surrounded by retinal haemorrhage

during transport the eye should be covered with a pad or plastic shield.

Methods of correcting vision and risk of injury

Twenty-five percent of all sportspeople require some form of refractive correction and the method chosen may affect the type and severity of injury sustained. Spectacles are the simplest method of correcting vision, but they may cause damage to a player or his opponent if worn in the contact or racket sports. Soft contact lenses are useful in this situation as, although they may become dislodged during play, unlike rigid lenses or spectacles, they will not shatter and, therefore, do not compound any damage to an injured eye.

Refractive surgery has become increasingly popular with sportspeople as a permanent method of correcting vision. Radial keratotomy, or incisional surgery, which has fallen out of favour since the introduction of laser treatment, weakens the cornea with potentially disastrous consequences (*Figure 18.7*). Surface laser surgery (PRK), the most common refractive procedure in this country today, probably carries little or no increased risk to the eye as it does not significantly weaken the cornea. The increasingly popular intracorneal laser or LASIK (flap and zap) treatment is not compatible with contact or combat sports for six months to one year after treatment, as there is a risk of the superficial flap becoming dislodged and lost.

Sports associated with ocular trauma

There is a close relationship between the type of sport being played and the risk of ocular injury. Frequency of injury depends, to some extent, on regional and national popularity; baseball is the commonest cause of sports associated eye injury in America, hurling in Ireland and football in the UK. Sports which use rapidly moving balls, employ sticks and racquets or involve any degree of body contact carry a relatively high risk of injury in any country. Such sports include the racket sports (squash, tennis and badminton), soccer, rugby, cricket and hockey. The combat sports, such as boxing and karate, by their very nature comprise a very high risk group for serious eye injuries.

Prevention and protection

In view of the time and resources invested in the management of serious eye injuries, and the poor outcome from such injuries, prevention is a priority. Prevention of ocular injuries in sport falls into three main categories, taking into account the potential for eye injury:

1 Ensuring that the rules of play are in the interest of eye safety and safe play is encouraged by appropriate coaching and training;

2 Screening players to prevent those with ocular conditions that would put them at particular risk of ocular injury, or would render them visually handicapped if they were to be injured from participatng in the very high risk combat sports

3 Wearing protective eyewear.

A British standard for eye protectors for squash has recently been approved and the currently available well fitting eye protectors, made of clear, light polycarbonate material that is fog and scratch proof, have encouraged many players to wear them (*Figure 18.8*).

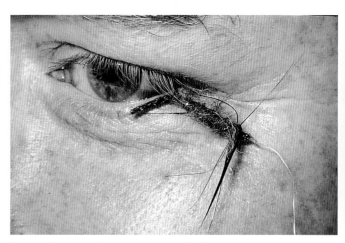

Figure 18.6 Penetrating injuries can be caused by fish hooks

Method of examination
- Check vision (count fingers, read signposts)
- Fields of vision to confrontation
- Examine the eye using a good light in a systematic fashion:
  —periorbital region
  —external eye—conjunctiva; cornea; sclera (assisted by using fluorescein drops)
  —intraocular contents—anterior chamber; pupil size, shape and reaction; posterior segment

Indicators of a serious injury
- Reduced vision
- Significant pain
- Hyphaema
- Abnormality of pupil shape or function
- Marked sub-conjunctival haemorrhage or swelling
- Chemical material has entered the eye
- Diplopia
- Arrange immediate referral to hospital if there is any doubt about the severity or nature of the injury, or if there is any

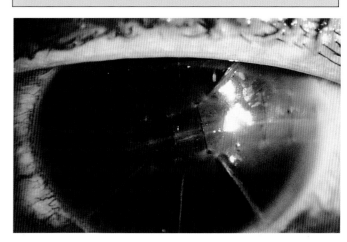

Figure 18.7 Repair of a cornea after incisional refractive surgery. The eye had been struck by a squash racket leading to rupture of one of the radial corneal refractive incisions that has been sutured

Contact lenses may be worn under these, or a prescription incorporated into the protective lenses to ensure good visual acuity.

Summary

- Eye injuries caused by sporting activities are often serious
- The most frequent sports in the UK to cause serious eye injury are football, the racket sports, rugby, and hockey
- When assessing an injury, always be aware of the circumstances and the type of injury suffered (for example, blunt, sharp), as this influences the type and extent of injury sustained
- Examine the eye systematically—bearing in mind that the lids should not be forced open
- Players need to see clearly to perform well—consider the method of correction for the 25% who have a refractive error as this may affect the injury sustained
- Refer immediately for a specialist opinion if a serious eye injury is suspected, or if the player proves difficult to examine
- Prevention is better than cure—always promote safe play and encourage the use of appropriate protective eye wear.

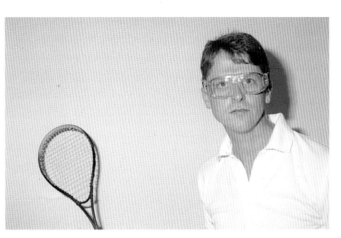

Figure 18.8: Eye protectors should be made of one piece polycarbonate and fixed firmly to the head

References

Vinger PF (1981) Sports eye injuries; a preventible disease. *Ophthalmol* **88**: 108–12

MacEwen CJ (1986) Sport-associated eye injuries: a casualty department survey. *Br J Ophthalmol* **71**: 701–5

Loran DFC, MacEwen CJ, eds (1995) *A Textbook of Sports Vision*. Butterworth Heinemann, Oxford

Zagelbaum BM, ed (1996) *Sports Ophthalmology*. Blackwell Science, Oxford

Acknowledgements

Figure 18.7 is produced with thanks to Dr G Crawford, Perth, Western Australia.

19 Risks of injury—an overview

David J Ball

Participation in sports, as with all other activities, carries with it a certain risk of injury. It is useful if not essential to have an idea of the magnitude of this risk and how it compares with other risks of life. The process of doing this is generally referred to as risk assessment. Risk assessment is not, however, an end in itself, but one of a number of tools that helps decision makers, who may be the individuals concerned or their advisers, decide on appropriate strategies. Other necessary information would typically include awareness of the benefits of the activity, the effectiveness of remedial measures and the associated difficulties of implementing them, including any costs.

The risk of fatal injuries

There are about 160 fatalities in sport and leisure related activities in England and Wales each year, about 10 per cent involving children under 15 years. About half of all the fatalities involve water related activities. In terms of numbers, this is a fairly modest contribution to the overall national toll of about 12 000 recorded accidental deaths per annum, the majority of which are attributable to road accidents, accidents at home, and workplace accidents.

A truer measure of risk takes account of how many individuals are exposed to the hazard in question and for how long, and a useful measure of risk in this regard is the Fatal Accident Rate (FAR), which refers to the number of fatalities per hundred million hours of exposure. FARs for adults in Britain range from unity or less for low risk sports, such as jogging, golf, and badminton, through two or three for contact sports, such as soccer, rugby, and hockey. Horse riding comes in at a FAR of about ten and water sports lie in a range up to about twenty. There is also a group of sports with considerably higher FARs, from 30 up to, perhaps, 200 or so. These include air sports, mountaineering activities, and motor sports.

Comparisons with other sectors

FARs for the riskiest sports are on a par with those found in the riskiest occupations, such as deep sea fishing and diving, and working on railway tracks. It would be the normal view that occupational risks at this level were as high as society would reasonably tolerate. The fact that individuals expose themselves to risks of this level, or higher, in sport is less contentious, although not uncontended, since it is generally regarded as voluntary. From time to time there are protests about such activities, but it seems unlikely that such risk-taking behaviour would ever be banned wholesale and it may well be that, for some personalities, therapeutic value or some other worth is found.

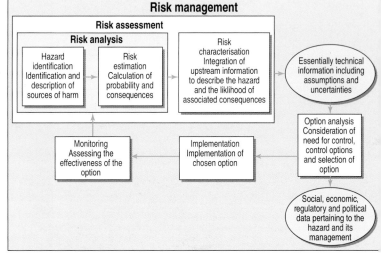

Figure 19.1 The relationship between risk assessment and risk management

Definitions

- Hazard—an object, activity or situation with the propensity to cause harm
- Risk—the probability that harm of a specified type may be realised as a result of exposure to a hazard
- Risk assessment—the process of assessing the magnitude of the risk and the consequences posed by a specified hazard
- Risk management—the process of making decisions about which remedial options, if any, to adopt. May also include the implementation and feedback stages

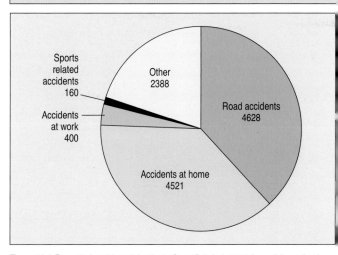

Figure 19.2 Recorded accidental deaths in Great Britain in 1992 by activity at the time of death

Aquatic sports and horse riding, with FARs of 10 to 20 or so, are on a par with travelling by car, while team sports with bats, balls, and sticks pose risks similar to those experienced by an elderly person at home. Lower risk sports, such as badminton, tennis, and golf, have FARs matching those of office workers or less.

Official guidance on the acceptability of FARs of whatever value has not been given, but, for illustrative purposes only, the Health and Safety Executive's workplace tolerability limit of 1 in 1000 per annum risk of death can be seen to be equivalent to a FAR of about 50 for a regular 40 hour working week (2000 hours per year). The higher risk sports exceed this criterion, as do a few higher risk occupations. The HSE tolerability limit for the public is 1 in 10 000 per annum and, assuming round the clock exposure in this case, the equivalent FAR is about unity. This is close to the FAR for ball/team sports, but ten times less than that of aquatic sports and horse riding, all of which are voluntary activities, whereas the HSE's criterion is based on circumstances of, to some degree, involuntary exposure.

Those levels of fatal risk deemed to be of trivial concern to the public are usually thought to be in the region of 1 in 100 000 per annum, to one in a million or less, and would be equivalent to FARs of 0.1 or lower. Lower risk sports, such as golf, may attain this level.

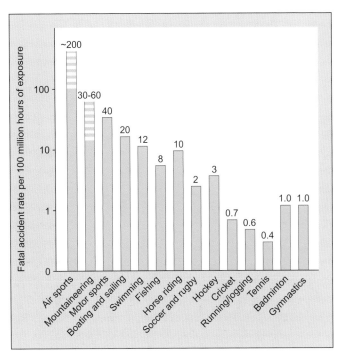

Figure 19.3 Estimated fatal accident rates per 100 million hours of exposure for selected sports

The risk of non-fatal injuries

It is believed that there are in the region of 20 million sports injuries each year in Britain, about half of which are attributable to soccer alone. Many of these injuries are slight, but the collective cost of treatment and lost production through time off work has been estimated as about £1 billion per annum. The most extensive data base on such injuries is the Leisure Accident Surveillance System (LASS) maintained by the Department of Trade and Industry. This provides data on attendances at hospital accident and emergency departments for sports related injuries. When combined with data on participation rates in specific sports, it is possible to estimate a

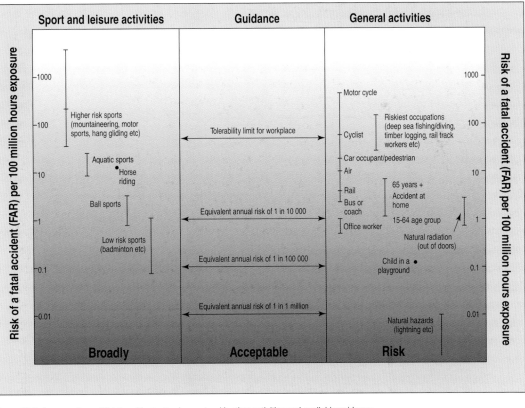

Figure 19.4: A comparison of fatal accident rates in sports with other activities and available guidance

Non-Fatal Accident Rate (NFAR) for each sport, thus producing a comparative ranking. NFARs are generally quoted in terms of the risk of a non-fatal injury per 100 000 hours of participation.

NFARs for more commonly played sports range downwards from about 300 for rugby to about unity for sports, such as golf, bowls, and table tennis. In between and at the top end lies soccer (130), closely followed by hockey and netball (80 to 90), with another group including cricket, basket ball, squash, and skiing coming in at 40.

Estimated risks of serious injuries per 100 000 hours of exposure to specified activities

Activity	Risk of occurrence per 100 000 hours		
	A&E attendance	Major injury	Over 3-day injury
Being at home (15 years and over)	2	-	-
Being at home (less than 15 years)	4	-	-
Playing in a playground	5	-	-
At the fairground	-	0.06	-
Driving a car	-	0.2	-
Riding on a motorcycle	-	7	-
Riding a bicycle	-	1	-
Working in a coal mine	-	0.3	2.4
Working in construction	-	0.2	1

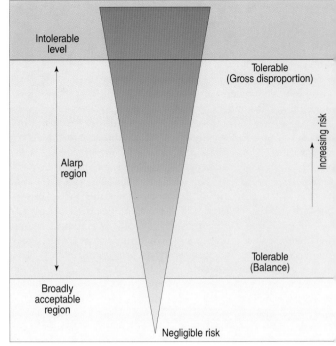

Figure 19.5 HSE guidance on the tolerability of risk. If risks are above an intolerable level the activity must normally cease. If risks are below a specified level they may be deemed as broadly acceptable. In between, risks must be reduced until As Low As Reasonably Practicable (ALARP)

Comparisons with other sectors

NFARs can be estimated for other types of activity, too, in order to provide a yardstick for comparison. For instance, the NFAR through simply being at home is two if you are 15 years old or more, and four if you are under 15 years. Interestingly, if NFARs are calculated for activities, such as working in a coal mine or on a construction site, they appear to be less than unity. Although the precision associated with these figures is low and strict comparisons are difficult, giving rise to considerable uncertainty, it seems that the risk of being injured at work, even in what were once regarded as comparatively hazardous occupations, is over 100 times less than that experienced during, say, a game of soccer.

Comments and observations

The full picture with regard to sports injuries is only partially revealed by this analysis because many non-fatal injuries are treated elsewhere than at hospital accident and emergency (A&E) departments. It has been estimated, however, that for every sports accident resulting in a fatality, there are 4000 A&E attendances, 25 000 seeking some other form of medical attention, and perhaps 100 000 who are self-treated or untreated.

One further important point about both the FAR and NFAR data described here is that they are based upon averages over the participating population, which consists primarily of younger age groups. Data on the risks that would be experienced by those most likely to benefit from

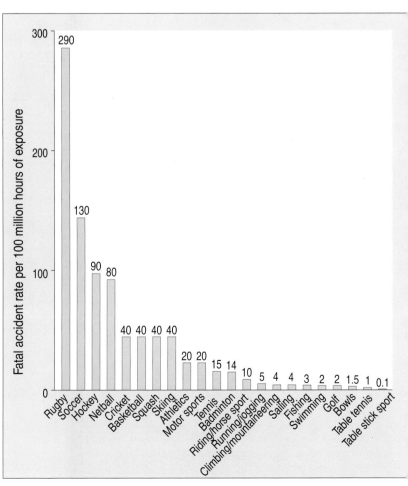

Figure 19.6 Estimated non-fatal accident rates, based on attendances at A&E departments, per 100 000 hours of exposure

more exercise, older men, females, and those who are inactive, are sparse.

Summary

The justifiable emphasis now placed upon public participation in sports and exercise, as a means of improving health and well-being and retaining independence in advanced age, should not lead to a neglect of the inevitable risks associated with these activities. Care is needed in the selection of exercise regimes, particularly for older persons and those previously inactive. Appropriate advice and facilities need to be available for would-be participants. Medical and rehabilitation services with specialist knowledge are necessary for the treatment of injuries that will, inevitably, arise. This should include recognition of the detrimental effects of immobilisation in elderly exercisers, who may require active treatment and rehabilitation with compensatory exercise therapy. It is also noted that there is a shortage of information on the risks of participation in sports by older participants, women and those previously inactive, and this needs to be addressed by further research.

References

Ball DJ (1998) The risks and benefits of sports and exercise. *Sports Exer Inj* Part 1 **4**: 3–9; Part 2 **4**: 74–9; Part 3 **4**: 174–82

Nicholl JP, Coleman P, Williams BT (1991) *A National Study of the Epidemiology of Exercise-related Injury and Illness*. The Sports Council, London

Nicholl JP, Coleman P, Williams BT (1995) The epidemiology of sports and exercise related injury in the United Kingdom. *Br J Sports Med* **29**(4): 232–8

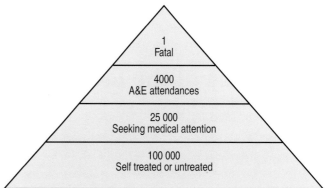

Figure 19.7 Accident triangle for sports accidents in the adult population

20 Injury of the face and jaw

K R Postlethwaite

Introduction

Although interpersonal violence is the most common cause of facial injury, sport, especially the contact sports, is also frequently associated with facial injury and recent studies have shown that the incidence is increasing.

The type of facial injury that can occur during sporting activities varies from simple cuts and abrasions, or minor dental injury to severely comminuted facial fractures. The latter may be associated with head and cervical spine injury; initial attention should also focus on the airway and the control of bleeding.

The injuries received often relate to the mechanism of injury and a good history from the patient or witnesses is important in guiding clinical examination. Accurate diagnosis will aid effective initial treatment and appropriate specialist referral.

Soft tissue injuries

Abrasions

Simple abrasions when contaminated require thorough cleaning and debridement to prevent infection and ugly pigmentation. This latter most commonly occurs when the abrasion is due to contact with a tarmacadum surface. Although simple debridement of superficial abrasions is possible, when large areas are involved, or where there is gross contamination, treatment may require local or sometimes general anaesthesia. Antibiotic prescription should also be considered (*Figure 20.1*).

Haematomas

These often settle spontaneously and rarely require drainage. However, blunt injury to the ear may result in a subperichondrial haematoma, which may result in cartilage deformity (cauliflower ear). Such haematomas should be drained either by needle aspiration, or a small incision and a pressure dressing carefully applied.

Nasal septal haematomas again require evacuation to prevent necrosis of the underlying cartilage.

Very occasionally large haematomas undergo liquefaction and exhibit fluctuance. If they fail to absorb after a period of 7–10 days then drainage can be helpful.

Lacerations

Again, these should be thoroughly debrided and antibiotics prescribed when there has been gross contamination. Thought should also be given to the need for tetanus prophylaxis.

When these are small, superficial and in uncomplicated areas of the face, accurate suturing under local anaesthesia using fine instruments and 5/0 or 6/0 monofilament nylon is appropriate. Very superficial wounds can sometimes be effectively treated with adhesive tapes (Steristrips).

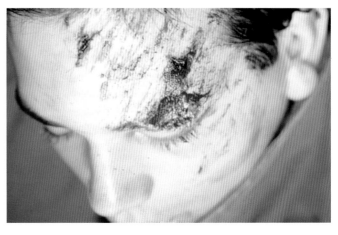

Figure 20.1 Extensive contaminated wound of forehead requiring thorough debridement and repair

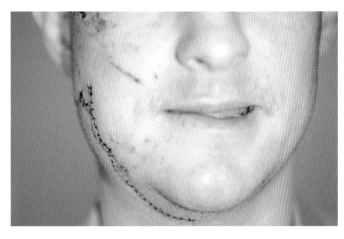

Figure 20.2 Laceration with severing of the cervical branch of the facial nerve

Lacerations requiring specialist referral

- Lacerations involving the lip vermilion, eyelids, and lacrimal apparatus
- Be aware of nerve injuries; check facial nerve function
- Parotid duct injury
- Where there is tissue loss or full thickness laceration of the lips
- Lacerations involving the cartilage of the ear or nose
- Intraoral mucosal lacerations

Deeper lacerations will require resorbable subcutaneous sutures, such as Polyglactin (Vicryl), to approximate the skin edges prior to the placement of skin sutures. Skin sutures can be covered in a polyantibiotic ointment (Chloramycetin or Polyfax), to prevent infection and to aid their removal at five to seven days.

Care should be taken with small puncture wounds, which may represent the entry point of a foreign body and will, therefore, require radiographic examination and possibly exploration.

It is important to check facial nerve function as lacerations involving sectioning of nerve branches should be urgently referred for microsurgical repair. This should be done systematically by asking the patient to look upwards or frown (frontalis branch), screw up the eyes (zygomatico-temporal), twitch the nose (buccal), and purse the lips (mandibular and cervical) (*Figure 20.2*).

Shaving the eyebrow prior to suturing of lacerations is not recommended as it can lead to misalignment and also problems of regrowth.

Intraoral lacerations can be difficult to suture due to problems of adequate access and are probably best referred to a maxillofacial unit.

Dental injury

Injury to the mouth may cause soft tissue injury and can often be associated with dental injury, teeth may be fractured, mobilised, subluxed, or avulsed.

Fracturing of the teeth may involve exposure of the sensitive dentine or dental pulp, which can be extremely sensitive and painful. Such teeth require appropriate dressing by a dental surgeon.

Mobilised teeth require splinting and thorough dental evaluation to exclude fracture of the root and to monitor vitality.

Subluxation (displacement) of teeth requires repositioning usually under local anaesthesia and splinting for 7–10 days.

Avulsed teeth may be successfully reimplanted although inappropriate first aid will adversely affect the prognosis; *success depends on correct initial treatment*.

Prevention of dental injury by the use of correctly fitted mouth guards should be mandatory in all contact sports.

Maxillofacial fractures

Such injuries should always be suspected when there has been any facial trauma. If there is any doubt, the referral for specialist advice should be made. Be aware that facial fractures may be associated with head and cervical spine injury (*Figure 20.3*).

The facial skeleton is divided into thirds (*Figure 20.4*) to aid systematic examination. Fractures of the nasal bones, cheekbone (zygoma), and mandible are the most common facial bony injury occurring in sport.

A general examination of the face should be carried out and should include a visual inspection, looking for deformity and asymmetry. This is aided by cleaning blood from the face. The facial skeleton should then be palpated, looking for areas of tenderness and possible bony steps most commonly felt around the orbital margins. Areas of facial paraesthesia may often indicate the presence of fractures due to damage of the various branches of the trigeminal nerve as they pass through bony foramina.

Nasal fractures

These may be associated with nasal bleeding that usually responds to local measures, such as the application of pressure, or occasionally nasal packing with Vaseline ribbon gauze. When there is prolonged or excessive bleeding, this may indicate more

Management of avulsed teeth
• If the tooth is successfully retrieved, hold the crown, **not** the root, to avoid damaging the periodontal ligament remnants
• Gently wash the tooth under cold tap water and, if possible, replace in the socket and retain it in this position by gently biting on a gauze or clean handkerchief
• If this is not possible, or when there is danger of inhalation, then transport the tooth in milk or isotonic fluid if this is available
• When avulsed teeth or fragments are not accounted for, and when there has been loss of consciousness, then the possibility of inhalation should be excluded by chest X-ray
• Refer for further specialist treatment

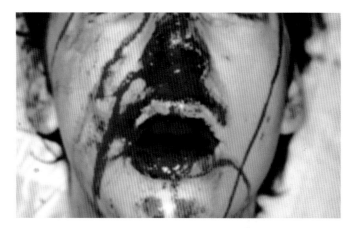

Figure 20.3 Patient with mid-face facial fractures; there was mobility of the maxilla

extensive bony injury. On occasions Foley catheters or Brighton's Balloons may be required as postnasal packs.

When seen immediately following the injury, deformity of the nose may be apparent but the rapid onset of swelling often masks this. Surgical treatment usually involves a closed manipulation of the fracture and application of a nasal splint. This treatment may be carried out immediately, but is often delayed for 7–10 days to allow swelling to settle. In some instances, late surgical intervention is indicated to correct deviation of the septal cartilage that is fractured and deviated, causing blockage of the nasal airway.

Zygomatic (cheekbone) fractures

Fractures of the zygomatic bones result in flattening of the affected side and facial asymmetry that is, again, often masked by swelling. Injury to the infraorbital nerve causing a characteristic area of facial numbness invariably occurs with fractures involving the zygomatic body (*Figure 20.5*).

As the zygoma forms both the lateral and inferior orbital walls, there is often associated injury to the eye and the periorbital tissues. The most frequent features seen are subconjunctival ecchymosis, blurring of vision, or diplopia. When the zygomatic

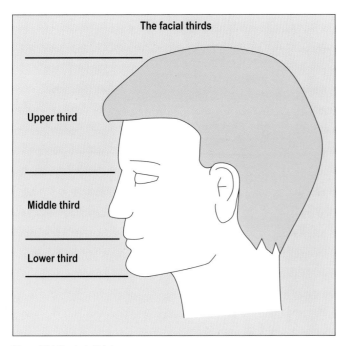

Figure 20.4 The facial thirds

The facial thirds

Upper third

Middle third

Lower third

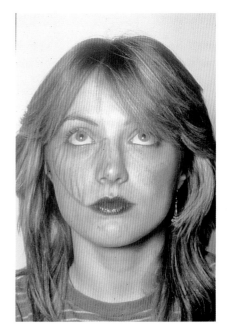

Figure 20.5 Area of numbness associated with infra-orbital nerve injury

arch is fractured there may be limitation of mouth opening due to the depressed arch impinging on the underlying temporalis muscle at its insertion to the coronoid process of the mandible.

Radiographic evaluation is carried out with occipitomental and submentovertex views to confirm the presence of a fracture, and degree of displacement.

Treatment involves reduction and internal fixation with small bone plates (*Figures 20.6 and 20.7*).

Internal orbital fractures

These are more commonly known as blow out fractures and usually involve the orbital floor and occasionally the medial wall (*Figure 20.8*). A blow out fracture should be suspected in any injury that involves a blow to the orbital area. They may be difficult to diagnose clinically and are commonly missed. The main features seen are diplopia, with "tethering" of the affected eye, usually to upward or lateral gaze, together with paraesthesia as a result of injury to the infraorbital nerve in its bony canal (*Figure 20.9*). A sunken appearance (enophthalmos) of the eye may be a late feature, but is often initially masked by periorbital swelling.

Investigation usually involves a CT scan, which, as well as confirming the fracture, provides information as to the site and extent of the defect (*Figure 20.10*).

Treatment

All cases should undergo maxillofacial and ophthalmic assessment prior to treatment, which may involve freeing of the trapped tissue and grafting of the defect to restore the contour of the orbit.

Mandibular fractures

The mandible is a horseshoe-shaped bone and fractures often occur bilaterally. They also occur at points of weakness, the condylar neck being the most common site. Pain and difficulty in occluding the teeth are an indication of mandibular fracture. Due to damage to the mandibular nerve within its bony canal, paraesthesia of the lower lip on the affected side is often seen.

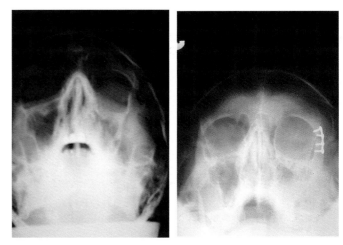

Figure 20.6 Depressed fracture of the left zygoma

Figure 20.7 Reduction and internal fixation of fracture

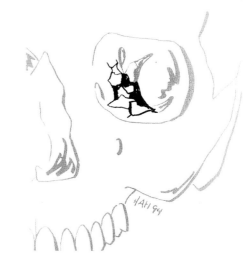

Figure 20.8 Blowout fracture involving medial and inferior orbital walls

Bony steps are not easily palpable extraorally apart from grossly displaced fractures. However, intraoral examination may be more helpful in revealing obvious steps in the lower dental arch or a deranged bite, (*Figure 20.11*) together with mucosal bruising and lacerations.

Treatment usually involves open reduction and internal fixation with small plates applied to the bone surface, most commonly via an intraoral approach.

Fractures of the middle third of face

Middle third facial fractures are usually seen following high velocity injuries or, on occasions, particularly violent assaults, they are not commonly seen following sporting injury, but should always be considered in trauma to the face. They should be suspected especially when there is derangement of the dental occlusion.

Summary

Soft tissue injury

- Facial and intraoral lacerations may require specialist referral
- Be aware of underlying nerve injuries (check facial nerve function).

Dental injury

- If the tooth is successfully retrieved and complete, hold the crown, NOT the root, to avoid damaging the periodontal ligament remnants. The earliest replacement in the socket is vital to success
- If required, transport should only be in an isotonic solution if available, milk, or the patient's own saliva.

Facial bony injury

- In all facial trauma with or without significant soft tissue injury, underlying bony injury should always be suspected with early referral for specialist advice if in any doubt
- Following such injury, it is recommended that contact sport should be avoided for a period of 6–8 weeks.

References

Crow R (1991) Diagnosis and management of sports-related injuries to the face. *Dental Clin N Am* **35**: 719–32

Emshoff R *et al* (1997) Trends in the incidence and cause of sport-related mandibular fractures. *J Oral Maxillofac Surg* **55**: 585–92

Rowe NL, Williams JW eds (1994) *Maxillofacial Injuries.* Churchill Livingstone, Edinburgh

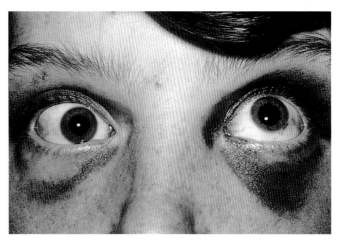

Figure 20.9 This patient with diplopia demonstrates tethering of the right eye to upward gaze, indicating a blowout fracture

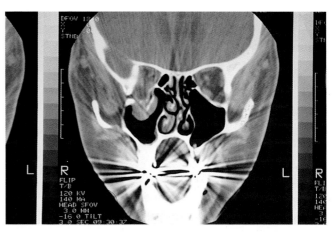

Figure 20.10 Coronal CT scan confirms a blowout fracture of the right orbital floor with prolapse of tissue from the orbit into the underlying maxillary sinus

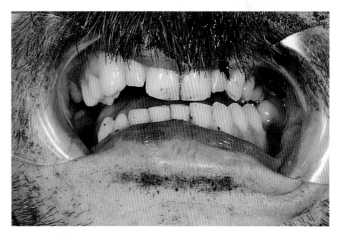

Figure 20.11 Patient with displaced middle third facial fracture and associated malocclusion (deranged bite)

21 Physiotherapy, sports injury, and the reacquisition of fitness

N Matthews

Introduction

One of the primary aims of the sports medicine professional is to create as safe an environment as possible for the athlete. However, "Sport for all" means injuries for all (McNab, 1991) and these injuries can occur as a result of trauma, overuse, or environmental factors. The majority of sports injuries are non-serious musculoskeletal lesions and complete recovery through rest and carefully planned rehabilitation is normal. However, whatever the cause of the injury, the physical capacity of the athlete is in some way diminished and recovery should not be left to chance. Rehabilitation programmes must be planned, positive, and dynamic.

Generally, a physiotherapist specialising in sports injuries has a well motivated, enthusiastic patient who will adhere to a set rehabilitative regime. However, acutely injured athletes must understand the importance that rest plays in the rehabilitative process and should be encouraged not to rush the rehabilitative process and thus hamper their long-term future.

Within a sporting institution the physiotherapist works within a multi-disciplinary team consisting of the coach, team manager, sports scientists and medical staff. The physiotherapist is nearly always the first member of this team to assess an injured individual, often while the person is still on the field of play. During this first assessment, a decision must be made upon the nature and severity of the injury and what immediate management to take. Initial first aid and management techniques may have a substantial bearing on the course and ultimate outcome of the rehabilitative process.

Whether directing rehabilitation alone or working with other members of the team, it should be remembered that the most important member of the team is the injured athlete and a successful rehabilitation requires communication, cooperation and coordination throughout the team.

Medical referrals do not always accompany the patient to the clinics and quite often it is the physiotherapist who makes the onward referral of the injured athlete for further medical investigation or treatment as is required.

The treatment aim of the physiotherapist is to restore the functional status of the athlete. This process must encompass not only the physical, but also the psychosocial aspects of any injury. Athletes are keen to return to the sporting arena and physiotherapists have to be sensitive and sympathetic to their emotional needs.

Rehabilitation

For a speedy return to the sporting arena treatment must initially be directed towards the injured area, pain should be controlled and unstable joints and fractures should be supported. As healing

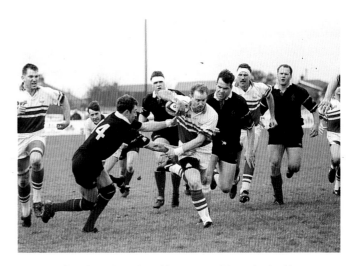

Figure 21.1 One of the primary alms of the sports medicine professional is to create as safe environment as possible for the athlete.

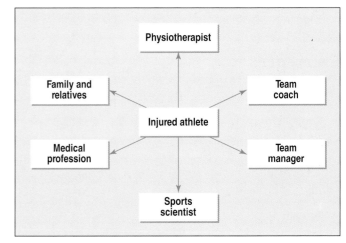

Figure 21.2 The injured athlete and the 'team'

The three 'C's of rehabilitation
- Communication
- Cooperation
- Coordination

Without communication, cooperation, and coordination, chaos will ensue

progresses and repair takes place it is important that the therapist safely progresses the rehabilitation to meet predetermined short-term goals. The design of any rehabilitation programme should protect the injured area and reduce pain. Where possible, joint range and muscle length should be maintained as should basic strength and muscle endurance. During rehabilitation, it may be necessary to re-establish neuromuscular function before the injured athlete is progressed to the final stages of rehabilitation and allowed back into the sporting arena.

Successful rehabilitation depends upon normal injury management principles. Initially, the problem must be assessed, evaluated, and given a diagnostic title. Then, in conjunction with the injured athlete, realistic short- and long-term objectives should be set. To achieve these objectives a viable treatment plan should be constructed. The actual rehabilitation should be a process of constant monitoring, reassessment, and further goal setting.

Exercise therapy

Therapeutic exercise is the mainstay of sports injury management. Accurate remedial exercises need to be learned by the injured athlete in order to preserve joint range of motion and muscular strength. In order to achieve this, there are innumerable exercises that can be employed, limited only by the imagination of the physiotherapist.

Muscular strength and endurance
Strengthening exercises should include isometric contractions (contraction without movement) and progressive resistive isotonic contractions (constant load throughout movement). Both concentric and eccentric exercises should be employed throughout the rehabilitation schedule. Manual techniques such as proprioceptive neuromuscular facilitation (PNF) can be used to increase both strength and joint range. Isokinetic exercise can be used if the equipment is available.

Stretching
A traumatically injured joint may heal with a reduced range of motion. To combat this an athlete should use specific stretching exercises prescribed by the physiotherapist to stretch the shortened structures involved. There are many forms of stretching and a multitude of different exercises, but there are certain basic guide lines and precautions that should be incorporated into a correct stretching programme.

Cardiovascular fitness
Alongside the remedial/therapeutic exercise regime, an alternative fitness schedule may have to be set out for the injured athlete in order to maintain cardiovascular fitness and muscular endurance.

Proprioceptive retraining
The ultimate goal of the rehabilitation programme is to reintroduce the athlete safely back to his or her chosen sport. For this reason the rehabilitative process does not stop when the injury has physiologically healed, but when the athlete is functionally able to take part in the chosen sport again. For this reason it is very important to prescribe proprioceptive retraining exercises. Proprioception encompasses the sensations of kinaesthesia and joint position sense and is controlled by joint, muscle, and cutaneous mechanoreceptors. Any retraining of these afferent deficits should result in enhanced kinaesthetic awareness and decrease the chances of re-injury. Afferent

---

Short-term aims of the rehabilitation programme
- pain control
- maintenance of joint range of motion (ROM)
- maintenance of basic strength
- re-establishment of correct neuromuscular function
- re-establishment of proprioception
- maintenance of cardiorespiratory fitness levels

The principles of rehabilitation
- Diagnosis
- Goal setting
- Treatment plan
- The rehabilitation programme

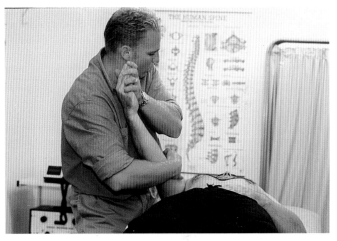

Figure 21.3 Manual PNF techniques can be used to increase both joint range and strength

Guidelines and precautions to stretching programmes
- Warm up using a slow jog or fast walk before stretching and keep warm throughout the session
- Muscles must be stretched beyond their normal ROM
- Stretch to the point of resistance not pain
- Avoid stretching joint in directions in which the joints do not naturally move
- Stretch slowly and with control; breathe normally
- For optimum effects you should stretch at least four times per week

Aims of stretching
- Improve flexibility of muscles
- Increase range of motion of joints
- Prevent injury
- Prevent post exercise stiffness and soreness

information from these structures, together with visual information, control joint stabilisation in differing positions. For example, an athlete with a damaged lateral ligament of the ankle may be completely at ease running on a flat surface in straight lines, but will not be able to cope in a sport that requires quick changes of direction and speed changes. A well structured rehabilitation regime will progress, when safe to do so, into replicating conditions experienced in the competitive arena. The staged interaction of the injured area with the external environment encountered while competing is essential if an injured athlete is to be pronounced fit to return to competitive sport.

Hydrotherapy

Exercise in the water can be a very beneficial form of exercise. It is especially useful during the early stages of rehabilitation when the injured athlete is unable to weight bear fully or move a joint against gravity. A purpose built hydrotherapy pool provides a warm relaxing environment in which an athlete can actively begin to mobilise injured structures safely through protective spasms. Water is also very useful for an athlete who is suffering from minor injuries that are aggravated by a normal training regime. For example, an athlete suffering from patella tendon tendinitis will aggravate the injury by running. In the water, with the use of buoyancy aids, the athlete will be able to the exercise without pounding already compromised structures

Massage

Massage can be used as an effective treatment technique or as an adjunct to injury prevention. Light massage techniques, such as effleurage and petrissage can help to improve muscle tone and circulation prior to exercise and help to reduce tightness following exercise. Light massage techniques may be used following injury to reduce pain and relieve muscle spasm. Stimulated mechanoreceptors within massaged structures may stimulate afferent nerves reducing pain via the pain gate theory.

Deep massage is frequently applied directly to the lesion in order to break down any adhesions or scar tissue. This is known as deep friction massage and is particularly useful in chronic lesions, especially tendinitis.

Therapeutic modalities

Therapeutic agents when used appropriately can be extremely useful tools in the rehabilitation of the injured athlete and work extremely well as adjuncts to exercise therapy.

Infrared modalities

Modalities which provide superficial heating or cooling of the tissues are known as infrared modalities. The use of cold is called cryotherapy and the superficial heating of tissues is called thermotherapy. Cold is most effective in the acute phases of the healing process, but both hot and cold are very effective in reducing the sensation of pain associated with injury.

Electrotherapeutic agents

There are many electrophysical agents available to the sports physiotherapist to help reduce pain and provide optimum healing conditions, so that normal movement can be resumed. The most commonly used is ultrasound, which can be used as a pulsed or continuous beam. The most significant effect of using continuous ultrasound is the production of heat in the underlying tissues, useful in chronic lesions. Pulsed ultrasound does not have any thermal effect. It is indicated for acute lesions where it has been shown to agitate tissue fluid, thus increasing the rate of phagocytosis. Ultrasound is also effective in reducing pain.

Methods of maintaining cardiovascular fitness
- Continuous activity
- Interval training
- Fartlek training
- Circuit training

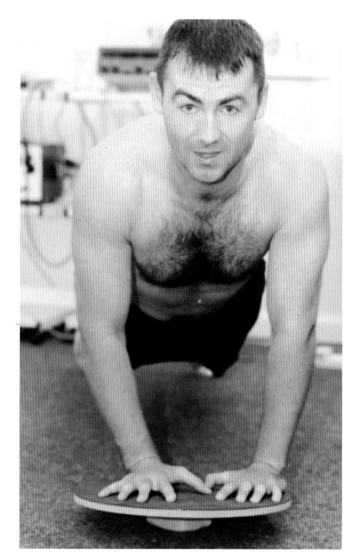

Figure 21.4 Proprioceptive training is vital if the athlete is to be pronounced fit for competitive sport

Aims of massage
- To relieve muscle spasm
- To reduce pain
- To facilitate swelling reduction
- To improve local muscle tone and circulation

Aims of manipulation and mobilisation
- To reduce pain
- To increase joint range of motion
- To restore functional range of motion

The prevention of sports injuries

Physical conditioning

As well as treating injuries caused by sport, sports physiotherapists have a role to play in injury prevention. They should ensure that athletes are adequately conditioned for the demands of the sport they are playing. It is also essential that athletes are fully aware of how to warm up and stretch before competing.

Support and strapping

In some cases, further injury to a joint can be prevented with the use of strapping and supports. This not only provides physical support, but also provides psychological support, relieves anxiety and boosts a player's confidence. A number of different materials and appliances are available to provide support for soft tissues and joints, the most common being neoprene system.

Protective equipment

Injuries can also be reduced by using protective equipment, such as padding and helmets. Generally, any protective equipment used must be light, durable and not restrict movement. It must not interfere with an athlete's ability to perform or be harmful to other competitors. Most importantly, it must be approved by the sports governing body.

Protective equipment should

- Be light and comfortable
- Allow full range of movement
- Not provide a risk of injury for other competitors
- Conform to the sports governing rules and regulations

Summary

Physiotherapists play a vital role in the rehabilitation of athletes competing at any level. Many injuries are caused by premature return to training and competition before the athlete is ready.

A positive attitude needs to be adopted by the physiotherapist and the athlete to ensure a speedy return to competition. Communication must be good at all levels to prevent misunderstandings. The sports physiotherapist's role encompasses not only prevention, treatment, and rehabilitation, but also includes friend, confidant, motivator, and agony aunt.

Physical effects of heat

- Increases cutaneous circulation
- Reduces muscle spasm
- Increases metabolic rate to optimum healing conditions
- Local anaesthesia

Heat provides an alternative treatment to ice, it is particularly useful in the sub-acute phase of injury

---

Physical effects of cold therapy

- Local anaesthesia
- Decrease in local metabolic rate
- Changes in peripheral circulation

The use of ice in the treatment of soft tissue injuries is universal

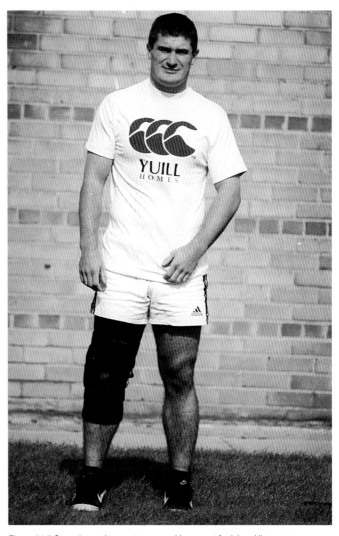

Figure 21.5 Strapping and supports can provide support for injured ligaments

22 Immediate management of severe injuries

I W R Anderson

Most forms of sport and exercise carry a risk of injury whether in the "serious" sportsperson or those in the pursuit of fitness or simply fun. An over-riding principle in the management of major injury in sport and exercise is primary prevention by meticulous attention to safety and avoidance of risk.

An essential requirement of all health care workers and others involved in sport and exercise is early recognition of possible serious injury and rapid, appropriate life-saving intervention. In the main, this usually involves fairly simple techniques and procedures. Just as in sport, skill in the immediate management of serious injury depends on preparation and practice, without which performance is usually poor or even pitiful.

Training courses covering pre-hospital and early hospital trauma care are available from respected postgraduate organisations, faculties, and colleges within the United Kingdom.

The immediate management of life-threatening injury has five components (ABCs). Head injury management has been detailed in a separate chapter.

It can be easy to be distracted from the ABCs by the visual impact of a dramatic limb injury. **Lives need to be saved before limbs** (*Figure 22.1*).

Airway (*Figures 22.2 and 22.3*)

The most common cause of airway obstruction is impairment in conscious level due to a head injury. Facial injuries, whether soft tissue or associated with underlying facial fractures, can cause mechanical obstruction to the airway, as can the accumulation of blood and vomitus.

Basic airway techniques, using either an oropharyngeal or nasopharyngeal airway with suction where appropriate, can convert a compromised airway to a patent airway. **All trauma patients are potentially hypoxic**.

- **All trauma patients need supplemental oxygen**

Advanced airway techniques can be lethal in the hands of the inexperienced who must be reassured that it is safe to fall back on basic techniques until additional expertise can be summoned.

Cervical spine

All patients who have sustained blunt trauma above the clavicle, especially those with an impaired level of consciousness, have not only a compromised airway, but also, more sinister, a potentially underlying cervical spine injury. Only in the following circumstances can a cervical spine injury be reasonably excluded:

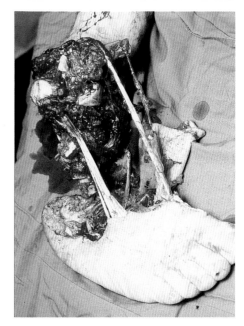

Figure 22.1

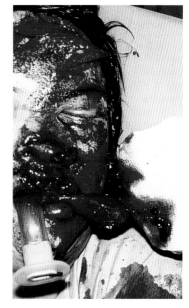

Figure 22.2

All other patients require cervical spine protection with the application of an appropriately sized commercial semi-rigid collar and in all patients other than those who are 'thrashers', the application of neck bolsters or sandbags and tape applied to anchor both forehead and chin.

Breathing

The following five conditions can rapidly kill. Remember the patient must already have a patent airway

Tension pneumothorax

A patient will be fighting for breath with impairment in chest wall movements, hyper resonance to percussion and absent breath sounds on the side of the tension. Both tracheal shift away from the side of the tension and cyanosis are late findings. Treatment requires rapid assessment of the clinical signs and the insertion of a wide-bore cannula above the third rib in the mid-clavicular line. The diagnosis of a tension pneumothorax must never wait for a chest X-ray and is always a clinical diagnosis requiring life-saving intervention. A tension pneumothorax can develop following a simple pneumothorax in a patient who is receiving artificial ventilation. Young patients are less tolerant of a tension pneumothorax in view of the mobility of the mediastinum. More definite care of the tension requires definite placement of an intercostal drain, through the fifth intercostal space anterior to the mid-axillary line, under aseptic conditions and through a short surgical incision, and subsequent surgical dissection through the tissues of the chest wall. The chest drain must be firmly secured and attached either to a valve device or under-water seal drain.

Massive haemothorax

Massive haemothorax may occur as a result of a severe force applied to the chest through blunt trauma or a penetrating wound.

A massive haemothorax is defined as some 1500 ml of blood in the chest cavity, which equates to almost a third of the circulating blood volume in a 70 kg adult. Treatment requires volume replacement and drainage.

Open pneumothorax

A sucking chest wound requires placement of a chest drain and coverage of the sucking defect as immediate measures.

Flail chest

Despite the dramatic appearance, the main problem is not damage to the chest wall, but damage to the underlying lungs with contusions causing ventilation perfusion mis-match.

Cardiac tamponade

This mimics the clinical signs of a tension pneumothorax without the findings on percussion or/and auscultation of the chest. A high index of suspicion should be raised in penetrating wounds between the nipples, in front, and shoulder blades, behind, the chest wall.

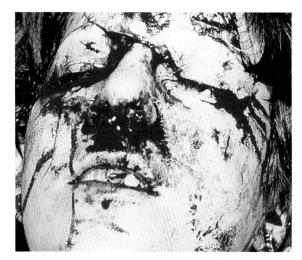

Figure 22.3

Circulation and control of bleeding

External sources of bleeding should be treated by direct pressure. Tourniquets have no place in the management of bleeding from wounds. An assessment of the situation can be made on clinical grounds with attention to conscious level, rate, and volume of peripheral pulses and the appearance of skin.

Those who regularly take part in sport and exercise are likely to have a low resting pulse rate and what in the community would be regarded as a normal pulse rate can, in such individuals, be a relative tachycardia. Compensatory mechanisms in fit individuals can result in the masking of the typical signs of blood loss until, at least, 30% of the blood volume has been depleted and before any of the normally associated signs of clinical shock are revealed.

There is little to be gained by aggressive volume replacement of blood loss at the scene, when transfer of a patient can be expedited within 15 minutes or so of injury. When transfer is, for any reason, likely to be delayed, particularly in the presence of an entrapment, significant blood loss requires **significant blood replacement** until arrangements can be made to allow the source of the bleeding to be identified and controlled, and this **always requires a surgeon with appropriate skills**.

Disability

Assessment of the conscious level by the Glasgow Coma Scale, together with pupil responses, has already been referred to in the chapter on head injury.

Exposure and environment

Always be aware of the possibility of hypothermia in the injured and the continuing dangers in the environment, both to those already injured and those in attendance.

Abdominal trauma *(Figure 22.4)*

The diagnosis of blunt abdominal trauma can be extremely difficult. Due attention must be paid to the mechanism of injury, particularly the possibility of a high-energy transfer, either as a result of a fall or a rapid acceleration/deceleration injury. Clinical signs of abdominal trauma can be masked in the presence of an underlying spinal cord injury with or without a head injury. Bruising and abrasions over the front, back, or sides of the abdomen may be useful pointers, as may the presence of bruising in the perineum or blood at the external urinary meatus.

Closed lower right-sided rib fractures may be a pointer to underlying liver injury and, so, too, can closed lower left-sided rib fractures to underlying splenic injury. The tissue diagnosis of the abdominal injury is not important, rather, it is important to realise that there is an underlying abdominal injury, no matter which organ is damaged and to arrange for the patient to be assessed by a surgeon.

Penetrating injuries to the lower chest may involve the upper abdominal cavity and vice versa. Blunt or penetrating wounds to the back, particularly to the flanks, will only be diagnosed when the patient is safely log-rolled to allow visual inspection of that part of the body.

Retroperitoneal injuries are frequently overlooked due to the absence of abdominal findings and require a high index of suspicion, given knowledge of the mechanism of injury.

All patients with abdominal pain following a sports injury require to be reviewed by a skilled Clinician before being given a clean bill of health.

Pelvic injury *(Figure 22.5)*

Pelvic fractures bleed profusely. Clinical signs of a pelvic fracture may well be subtle, but should be suspected given knowledge of the mechanism of injury, particularly that which involves high-energy transfer. The pelvis should be gently examined, but crepitus, if elicited, must never be repeated. Open pelvic fractures require urgent orthopaedic intervention to close the pelvic ring by the application of an external fixation device. In the meantime, sandbags can be placed on either side of the pelvis behind the hips, in a bid to control the pelvic diameter and prevent excessive movement during transfer to hospital.

Musculoskeletal injury *(Figure 22.6)*

Injuries to the limbs frequently maim, but rarely kill. They may distract attention from more serious threats to life that would be diagnosed by attention to the ABCs.

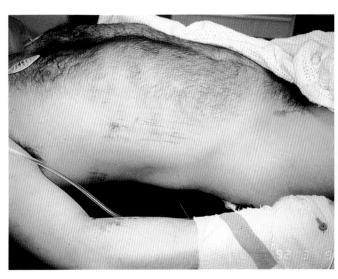

Figure 22.4 Abdominal trauma

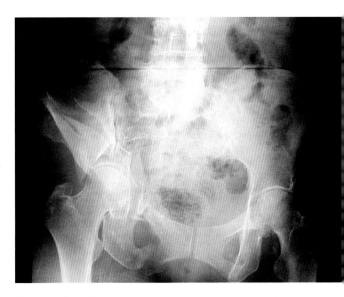

Figure 22.5 Pelvic injury

Limbs should be examined by:

- Look
- Feel
- Move
- X-rays

In a mechanism of injury involving a high-energy transfer, patients who have sustained upper and lower limb injuries may well have suffered serious injury to the chest, abdomen, spine, or pelvis.

Both the rate of bleeding and the level of pain in fractures may be improved by splintage of the limb in as anatomical a position as possible.

Care must be taken to evaluate the circulation and nerve supply to each injured limb. Bleeding from a limb should be controlled initially by direct pressure only.

Crushing injuries to limbs can cause serious systemic complications due to traumatic rhabdomyolysis.

Acute impairment in limb circulation is a surgical emergency and requires rapid transfer to hospital.

Open fractures should be covered with a moist dressing and splinted appropriately—once covered the dressing should not be disturbed until prior to definitive care. Traumatic amputation of a limb is the most severe form of open fracture. The amputated part should be wrapped in moistened gauze, placed in a plastic bag and then must be transported, with the patient, in as cool an environment as possible, for example, with crushed ice.

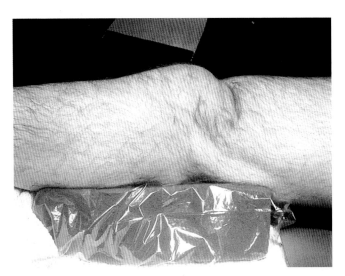

Figure 22.6 Musculoskeletal injury

Compartment syndrome

A pulse is usually present in compartment syndrome and the absence of a pulse is a very late sign in compartment syndrome.

The diagnosis of a compartment syndrome is made on clinical grounds with a high index of suspicion and demands urgent treatment to prevent permanent complications of ischaemic contracture.

The hallmarks of compartment syndrome in an injured limb are:
- Pain
- Paraesthesia
- Diminished power and sensation

Thermal injuries (*Figure 22.7*)

Burns

Facial burns with heat and/or smoke inhalation may cause rapid airways compromise.

The extent of body surface area burn can be estimated using the Rule of Nines. Partial thickness burns are red and exquisitely painful. Full thickness burns are leathery in appearance and non-painful. The burning process must be stopped by removing all clothing. Treatment of thermal injury is exactly the same as any other form of injury already discussed with due attention to the ABCs.

A useful first aid dressing for burns is the application of commercial kitchen cling film, which has the added bonus of giving some form of pain-relief.

Cold injury

Local hypothermia can result in freezing of local tissues, that is frostbite or non-freezing injury, for example, trench foot.

Systemic hypothermia can occur as a complication in patients with concomitant major injury. Treatment requires removal from the hostile environment, together with local or systemic re-warming techniques with due adherence to the principles of the ABCs.

Resuscitation in profound hypothermia may require active core re-warming in an intensive care or critical care environment.

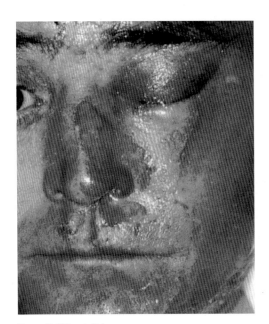

Figure 22.7 Thermal injury

Analgesia

Painful conditions always require appropriate pain relief and reassurance. Appropriate splintage of limb injuries can go some way towards relieving pain and an inhalational analgesic has a useful role

In serious injury, intravenous opioids are required, given in incremented dosages titrated against patient need and response.

Further reading

American College of Surgeons Committee on Trauma (1997) *Advanced Trauma Life Support Student Manual*. American College of Surgeons, Chicago

Anderson ID, Anderson IWR, Clifford P, *et al* (1997) Advanced trauma life support in the UK: 8 years on. *Br Med J Hosp Med* **57**: 272–3

Driscoll PA, Vincent CA (1992) Organising an efficient trauma team. *Injury* **23**: 107–10

Skinner D, Driscoll P, Earlam R (1996) *ABC of Major Trauma*. BMJ Publishing Group, London

23 Fluid balance during exercise

R J Maughan

Hard exercise is associated with a high rate of metabolic heat production and a rise in body temperature. Heat gained from the environment when the weather is warm adds to the heat load (*Figure 23.1*). Sweating during exercise is effective in limiting the rise in body temperature that occurs, and thus protects the athlete from the dangers of hyperthermia. The loss of water and electrolytes (salts) is a potential problem, and replacement of these is necessary to avoid the reduction in exercise capacity that results from dehydration. For a typical sedentary individual living in a temperate climate, about 2–3 litres of water is lost from the body by all routes each day. In hard exercise, sweat rates of 1–2 litres per hour are often seen and, in exceptional circumstances, a loss of 3 l/h may occur. The athlete training hard in a hot climate may need anything from 4–12 litres of water per day, depending on the training load and the sweating characteristics of the individual.

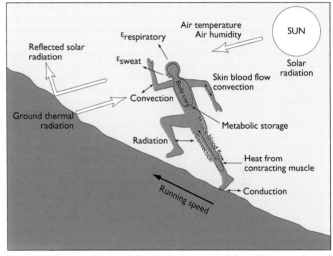

Figure 23.1 High rates of metabolic heat production must be balanced by an equal rate of heat loss to limit the rise in body temperature. In warm weather, when ambient temperature is equal to or greater than skin temperature, the only avenue of heat loss is by evaporation of sweat from the skin

Approximate average values for water loss (ml/day) from the body for sedentary adult men and women. With hard exercise in a hot environment, sweat rates may reach 3 litres per hour

	Men	Women
Urine	1400	1000
Expired air	320	320
Trancutaneous loss	530	280
Sweat loss	650	420
Faecal water	100	90
Total	3000	2110

In hot weather, the capacity for exercise is dramatically reduced (*Figure 23.2*) and a combination of high ambient temperature and humidity, together with dehydration is a major challenge. Preparation for such conditions requires an acclimatisation strategy and a fluid replacement plan. Acclimatisation requires repeated exposures to heat strain, and can be achieved by exercise in the heat for periods between 30 and 100 minutes per day. Adaptation begins after the first exposure and is largely complete after 10–12 sessions if these are carried out on a daily basis. Although athletes may be tempted to believe that the need for fluid replacement will decrease as they become adjusted to the heat, heat acclimatisation will actually increase the requirement for fluid replacement because of the enhanced sweating response. If dehydration is allowed to occur, the improved ability to tolerate heat that results from the acclimatisation process will be lost. There is no way of adapting to dehydration; attempting to do so is futile and dangerous.

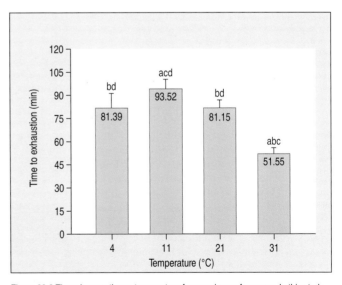

Figure 23.2 There is an optimum temperature for exercise performance. In this study, involving prolonged strenuous exercise on a cycle ergometer, the best performance was seen at an ambient temperature of 11°C; already at 21°C, performance time was significantly reduced

Drinking before exercise

It is important to begin each training session or competition fully hydrated. The idea that the body can adapt to exercise in the dehydrated state by deliberately restricting fluid intake is mistaken. If this is attempted, the quality of the training session is reduced. This is one situation where, just because it feels harder to train, it does not mean that it is doing more good. Attempts to train while dehydrated will greatly increase the risk of heat exhaustion and of life-threatening heat stroke. Every effort should be made to take fluids before training, and the best fluid to take at this time is probably one of the commercially available sports drinks. The major difference between these drinks is taste, and athletes should experiment with different drinks and with different flavours of each brand. It is important to find a product with a taste that is appealing. When the fluid requirement is as much as 8–10 litres of fluid per day, several different drinks or different flavours of the same drink may help to encourage consumption by providing some variety.

Monitoring of fluid status is important and athletes should learn to recognise the symptoms of dehydration. These include infrequent urination and the passing of small volumes of dark urine. Urine colour charts (*Figure 23.3*) are helpful in encouraging athletes to ensure adequate fluid intake. Many of the symptoms of jet lag are similar to those of mild dehydration—these include fatigue, headache and insomnia—and where these symptoms are present it may be wise to increase fluid intake.

Athletes in weight category or weight-sensitive sports need to be careful with their drinking strategy. Most of the sports drinks contain about 6–7% carbohydrate, so 1 litre will give 60–70 grams of carbohydrate, which adds up to about 250–300 calories. Drinking 5 litres of a sports drink can give up to 1500 calories—this may be more than half the total daily energy needs of many athletes. Most popular soft drinks contain even more: an athlete drinking 10 litres of cola per day will get over 4000 calories, before even beginning to eat any solid food. For the well fed, well rested athlete, water or low-energy drinks may be the best choice in this situation.

Drinking during exercise

Fluid intake during exercise is aimed at countering the effects of dehydration and can also provide a source of energy, usually in the form of carbohydrate. Recent results show that the benefits of providing fluid and carbohydrate are independent and additive. In some sports, there are limited opportunities for fluid intake during competition because of the nature of the event, or because of restrictions imposed by the rules. In most situations, however, voluntary intake is insufficient to match losses and increasing intake would be likely to be beneficial (*Figure 23.4*).

If the exercise period is short, there is no time for drinks ingested to be absorbed, and even when exercise time stretches to 1 hour or more, it is important that ingested fluids are available quickly. The rate at which fluids can be replaced is limited by the rate of gastric emptying and of intestinal absorption of water and nutrients. There are large individual differences in the rate at which these processes occur, so each athlete must establish his or her own best drinking pattern.

Figure 23.4 Players in games, such as football, must take advantage of available opportunities to replace sweat losses in training as well as in competition: fluid replacement is necessary even when these games are played in cool environments

Figure 23.3 Athletes should be encouraged to monitor urine colour: darker colours indicate an inadequate fluid intake. This method is just as reliable as more sophisticated measurements, such as osmolality or conductivity. Reproduced from Urinary Indices of Hydration Status. Int J Sport Nutrition 1994; **4**: 265–790

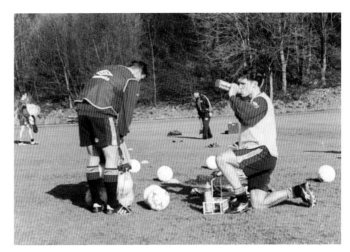

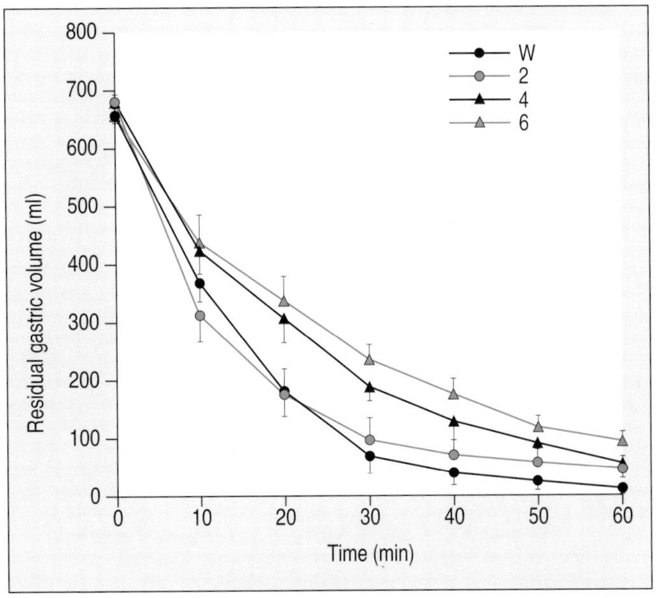

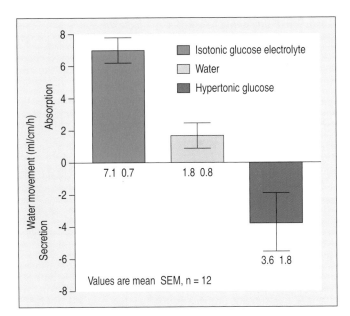

Figure 23.5 The rate of gastric emptying of liquids falls rapidly as the volume in the stomach falls, and emptying is slowed in proportion to the amount of carbohydrate present: this figure compares emptying rates of water, 2%, 4%, and 6% glucose solutions. Keeping the gastric volume high by repeated drinking is necessary to optimise the replacement of fluids

Factors promoting recovery after prolonged exercise

Recovery of muscle glycogen stores:
   Ingestion of carbohydrate as soon as possible after the end of exercise
   100–200 g should be ingested in the first 2 hours after exercise
   A high carbohydrate diet (5–10 g CHO/kg body weight/day) should be consumed
Restoration of fluid balance:
   The volume of fluid ingested should be at least 1.5 times the volume of sweat lost
   Electrolyte content of drinks or food should be sufficient to replace sweat electrolyte loss
   Sodium is the major electrolyte to be replaced

Gastric emptying of liquids is influenced by a number of factors, the most important of which are the volume of fluid in the stomach and the energy density of the drink (*Figure 23.5*). To replace fluids quickly requires a high volume of fluid in the stomach. An initial large drink followed by regular drinking of small volumes is the best way to keep the stomach topped up. The feeling of a full stomach during exercise is uncomfortable in the early stages, but the body adapts in time if the athlete persists. The time to adapt is in training; it is too late on competition day. This is also the time to experiment with different drinks to establish individual taste preference. Athletes who do not experiment with different strategies in training are unlikely to develop an optimum drinking strategy for competition.

Water absorption occurs mainly in the upper part of the small intestine and depends on osmotic gradients. Hypotonic drinks give the fastest rates of water absorption, but because active absorption of glucose and sodium promotes water absorption, dilute glucose-electrolyte solutions are more effective than plain water (*Figure 23.6*). Strongly hypertonic solutions (such as fruit juices or cola type drinks) cause a net secretion of water into the intestine. Although the water is eventually absorbed in the distal part of the intestine, this delay is not helpful when speed of fluid replacement is critical.

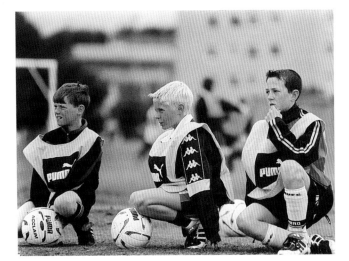

Figure 23.6 Isotonic glucose-electrolyte drinks are more effective than plain water in stimulating water absorption in the small intestine. Concentrated solutions with a high osmolality stimulate a net secretion of water

Types of drinks

Drinks with a low sugar content (about 2–4%, or 20–40 grams per litre) will not supply much energy, but if they are hypotonic and have a high sodium content (about 40–60 mmol/l, equivalent to about 1–1.5 grams per litre) they will give the fastest water replacement. The fastest rate of energy supply is achieved with high sugar concentrations (15–20%, 150–200 grams per litre, or even more), but this limits the rate at which water is absorbed. Electrolyte replacement is not normally a high priority during exercise, but may become important in very prolonged events (4 hours or more) where sweat losses are large and where there is no

Figure 23.7 Young athletes will not voluntarily replace fluids in sufficient volume to replace sweat losses and must be encouraged to drink more

opportunity to take solid food. The balance between the demands for water, carbohydrate and electrolyte replacement influences the choice of drink. Most of the commercially available sports drinks are a compromise aimed at providing both water and carbohydrate. Athletes and teams should discuss their individual requirements with a qualified sports nutritionist or dietitian to identify the most appropriate approach.

Men and women respond similarly to exercise in the heat and the variation between individuals outweighs any gender difference. The sensation of thirst does not normally promote sufficient intake to match losses and some degree of dehydration is normally observed, so drinks that taste good and encourage consumption should be chosen. Children are particularly susceptible to problems in the heat and must be encouraged to drink (*Figure 23.7*).

Drinking after exercise

Recovery after exercise requires replacement of the energy stores (especially muscle and liver glycogen) and restoration of water and electrolyte balance. Glycogen replacement is fastest if carbohydrate is consumed immediately after exercise, and can be achieved by eating or drinking 50–100 g of carbohydrate within the first 1–2 hours. Taking high carbohydrate drinks or eating high carbohydrate foods (confectionery, sweet biscuits, etc) with water are equally effective. Where sweat losses are high, large volumes of fluid should be consumed, and extra salt may usefully be added to the first meal. A change in the appetite for salt normally ensures an adequate intake without taking salt tablets. If no solid food is taken before the next training session, or the next round of events, some salt should be present in the fluids consumed and the sports drinks help to provide this. If the electrolytes lost in sweat are not replaced, the ingested fluid is not retained and a diuretic response is invoked, preventing full recovery even when large volumes of fluid are ingested. As a guide, the volume of fluid ingested should be at least 1.5 times the volume of sweat lost. The sweat loss can be estimated from the change in body weight: a loss of 1 kg of body weight means a sweat loss of 1 litre (*Figure 23.8*).

Drinks with a high alcohol content (spirits, wine, etc) have a strong diuretic effect, as does caffeine in tea and coffee—these drinks stimulate urine output and delay the rehydration process. Drinks with a high carbonation level may cause problems and should form only a small part of the total fluid intake. The gas content leads to a feeling of stomach fullness and discomfort, which, in turn, inhibits further intake of drinks.

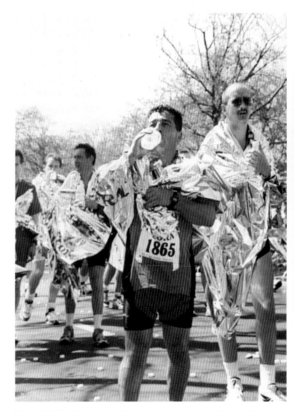

Figure 23.8 Rapid and complete replacement of sweat losses after exercise is an important part of the recovery process

Summary

- Fluid loss is greatly increased in the heat: daily fluid requirements may increase by 2–3 times normal
- Both dehydration and carbohydrate depletion impair performance
- An adequate intake of an appropriate fluid before, during (where appropriate) and after training and competition is essential for optimum performance
- Individuals must experiment in training to establish the most effective fluid replacement strategy

Acknowledgements

Figure 23.2: Reproduced from: Galloway SDR, Maughan RJ (1997) Effects of ambient temperature on the capacity to perform prolonged cycle exercise in man. *Med Sci Sports Ex* **29**: 1240–9

Figure 23.3: Reproduced with permission from: Armstrong *et al* (1994) Urinary indices of hydration status. *Int J Sport Nutr* **4**: 265–79

Figure 23.5: Reproduced with permission from: Vist GE and Maughan RJ (1994) The effect of increasing glucose concentration on the rate of gastric emptying in man. *Med Sci Sports Ex* **26**: 1269–73

Figure 23.7: Photograph courtesy of R Besant

24 Benefits of exercise in health and disease

Patrick S Sharp

Obesity

Experience teaches that lack of regular exercise leads to weight gain, but it is remarkable how difficult this has been to prove in human experiments. Comparison of activity levels in school children has shown that the more obese subjects are less active, but also eat less. In adults results have been less clear, but show similar findings when submitted to meta-analysis. What is not clear from these studies is whether obesity is the cause or effect of reduced activity, but a small number of studies have demonstrated reduced activity at baseline in subjects with greatest subsequent weight gain.

An equally important question is whether increasing physical exercise results in weight loss? A number of studies have demonstrated weight reductions in the order of 0.1 kg/week with regular exercise programmes (*Figure 24.1*), although it should be noted that exercise will also increase fat free mass, and loss of adipose tissue will be considerably greater than the figures show. Far greater weight reduction in the order of 0.6 to 1.8 kg/week, has been shown with more strenuous exercise in studies of military recruits, although it is doubtful that most free living individuals could match this. It would not, therefore, be prudent to offer such figures to those planning to lose weight by exercise alone.

Much of the change in weight induced by exercise will be accounted for by increased energy expenditure exceeding intake, but there are a number of other theoretical considerations. Glycogen storage in skeletal muscle is one of the major limiting factors in prolonged exercise performance. One of the body's adaptations to regular exercise, therefore, is preservation of glycogen stores. This is achieved by a switch to fat combustion. This was elegantly shown in one leg endurance training on a bicycle ergometer. After six weeks training, there was a smaller release of lactate from the trained leg than from the untrained leg, and a larger percentage of energy consumption in the trained leg stemmed from the use of fat as an energy substrate. The mechanism is thought to relate to upregulation of oxidative enzymes. Studies utilising indirect calorimetry have confirmed this finding, demonstrating a reduced respiratory quotient in the exercise trained individual indicating greater reliance on fat oxidation (*Figure 24.2*).

Given that exercise alone can result in only modest reductions in body fat, the next obvious question to ask is whether exercise coupled with dietary restraint has any added advantage.

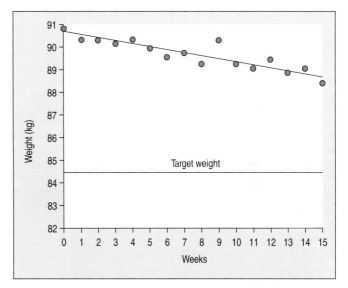

Figure 24.1 Example of weight loss achieved by individual cycling an average of one hour per day without any form of dietary restraint. The target weight will take many months to achieve

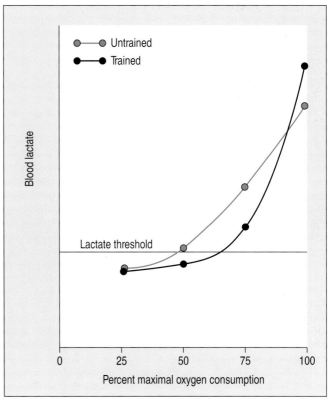

Figure 24.2 Increases in blood lactate concentration at different levels of exercise in trained and untrained individuals. The lactate threshold is that exercise level at which blood lactate rises steeply. Training increases the exercise capacity of the individual before reaching the lactate threshold and increases use of fatty acids as a fuel, thus conserving glycogen stores

As a starting point, it is important to note that, although extreme exercise may have a temporary anorectic effect, in the longer term, increased energy output is associated with increased intake. Dietary restraint would, therefore, need to be a conscious additional effort. Consumption of high energy drinks should be avoided since they are unnecessary in the casual exerciser. Studies of increased exercise and maintenance of dietary intake have shown considerable weight reductions, but it is interesting to note that the weight reductions are not as great as anticipated, most likely due to a reduction in metabolic rate associated with the relative energy restriction. Combinations of exercise and dietary restriction have not shown any attenuation of the reduction in metabolic rate caused by diet, but the addition of exercise does increase the contribution of fat loss, rather than muscle mass, to total weight reduction and it must be right to advocate exercise as part of a weight reducing regimen. In support of this is the consistent finding that a combination of diet and exercise is very much more successful in maintaining weight reduction than diet alone (*Figure 24.3*).

Diabetes

The beneficial effects of exercise in improving glycaemic control are many. Glucose uptake by many tissues, including muscle, the major consumer of glucose, is by facilitated diffusion. Glucose moves down a concentration gradient in a process involving a carrier molecule that transports hexoses across the cell membrane. This process is influenced by hormones and other intra and extracellular factors. Insulin is clearly the major hormonal factor. Following an acute bout of exercise, glucose uptake into muscle is stimulated. In part, this may be due to increased muscle blood flow and increased sensitivity to insulin, but may also relate to increased glucose transport in response to an increase in cytoplasmic calcium. Thus, exercise and insulin have an additive effect on glucose transport. As a point of clinical interest, the increased insulin sensitivity following exercise can last for 1–2 days, and together with depleted glycogen stores, can predispose to hypoglycaemia in insulin treated diabetics long after cessation of exercise.

The theoretical returns, therefore, are many for the subject with diabetes. In practice, in type I diabetes, these have been hard to demonstrate in the narrow terms of improvement in glycaemic control. This most probably arises from the difficulty in titrating the glucose and insulin intakes with exercise dose. If blood insulin levels are low at the onset of exercise, the result is hyperglycaemia that is beyond the capacity of increased peripheral utilisation. Production of counter-regulatory hormones increase lipid mobilisation and ketogenesis, all of which conspire to reduce exercise capacity. By contrast, high insulin levels at onset of exercise decrease hepatic glucose production and, together with increased peripheral utilisation, leads to profound hypo-glycaemia. Reduced fat mobilisation reduces lipid as a substrate, exacerbating the problem. Given this tightrope the insulin treated individual has to walk, it is not surprising that the benefits of exercise are hard to realise. Perhaps more encouraging are the results of studies looking at cardiovascular risk factors in subjects with type I diabetes, suggesting that a moderate exercise pro-gramme can reduce LDL cholesterol and raise HDL cholesterol by some 10–16%. With care and appropriate advice, there are virtually no sports which are closed to insulin treated individuals, and most studies indicate that in the absence of complications, exercise tolerance is normal.

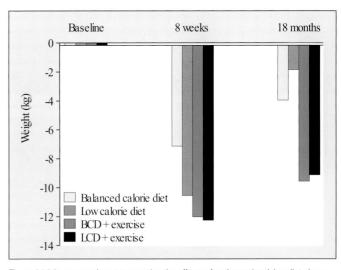

Figure 24.3 In an experiment to examine the effects of regimens involving diet alone, and diet plus exercise, those regimens which included exercise were more successful in maintaining weight loss than those that included diet alone (Adapted from Pavlou *et al*, *Am J Clin Nutr* 1989;**49**:1115–23)

Guidelines for exercise in insulin taking diabetic subjects

- Monitor glycaemia before, during (if possible), and after exercise
- Consume a snack of 15 to 40 g carbohydrates for every 30 to 60 minutes of intense exercise
- Intermediate acting insulin — reduce the dose by 30% if exercise can be predicted and is likely to be strenuous
- Short acting insulin — reduce the pre-exercise dose by 30–50% according to experience
- Use non-exercising sites for insulin injection
- Monitor blood glucose carefully for 24 hours after strenuous exercise

Guidelines for exercise in non-insulin dependent diabetes

- Seek a medical opinion before undertaking exercise, including a blood pressure check, ECG, lipid measurements, and assessment of glycaemic control
- Assess optimal exercise intensity according to one of the methods given below

Fortunately in type II diabetes, the situation is clearer and a reduction in HbA1 of 1–1.5% has been demonstrated. Provided glycaemic control is good, no special precautions need be taken, although it would be wise to be alert to the possibility of hypoglycaemia since this is commonly unrecognised by the tablet treated individual. It is also important to note that vascular disease is common in this group and a medical opinion may be required prior to undertaking an exercise programme to ensure fitness.

Hyperlipidaemia

The effects of exercise on lipid and lipoprotein metabolism are well known; active individuals have higher levels of HDL and HDL_2 cholesterol, and lower levels of VLDL and dense LDL cholesterol compared with sedentary individuals. Exercise increases the ability of muscle to take up and utilise free fatty acids and increases the activity of lipoprotein lipase, improving the efficiency of the cascade from VLDL to HDL and LDL cholesterol. It is difficult to separate the effects of exercise alone from the loss of body fat that accompanies exercise, but a number of well conducted trials suggest that the effects are separate and of similar order. This being the case, there is reason to expect that the effects may be additive. Nevertheless, most studies demonstrate reductions in cholesterol and triglyceride of only 0.1–0.3 mmol/l, and it is important to bear this in mind when prescribing exercise for hyperlipidaemia, notwithstanding that benefits extend beyond simple lipid changes (*Figure 24.4*).

Hypertension

Epidemiological and clinical studies have demonstrated an association between physical activity and lower blood pressure. As a therapeutic intervention, however, the use of exercise in lowering blood pressure has met with variable results. The majority of studies show a reduction in systolic and diastolic blood pressure in the order of 11 and 8 mmHg respectively, but rarely is the reduction sufficient to render study subjects normotensive. A significant minority of studies show no benefit of exercise on blood pressure, suggesting that there is a subgroup of hypertensive subjects who are resistant to exercise as a therapy. Nevertheless, despite variable results, exercise should be recommended to mildly hypertensive subjects in the context of reduction of cardiovascular risk, although this may not avoid the necessity to resort to pharmacological means of blood pressure reduction (*Figure 24.5*).

Cardiac rehabilitation

From the above discussion, it is apparent that exercise as a therapy has the potential to reduce cardiac risk factors in healthy individuals, and numerous studies attest to the fact that similar benefits in terms of weight reduction and improvement in lipid profiles can be achieved in subjects with known cardiac disease. There is understandable concern that exercise poses a particular risk in cardiac patients, but, properly prescribed, it is possible to achieve useful work rates in those with established heart disease. The current vogue for work-out in the gym has led to the publication of a body of literature suggesting that resistance work is safe, and even desirable, in this group.

Improvement in surrogate markers of risk in heart patients, while valuable, do not justify prescribing a theoretically hazardous

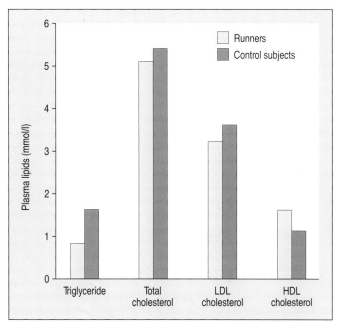

Figure 24.4 In a comparison of lipid levels in those who run regularly and control subjects, it was demonstrated that there was a beneficial effect on the lipid profile. Data for men are shown, but effects were similar in women (Adapted from Wood and Haskell, Lipids 1979;**14**:417)

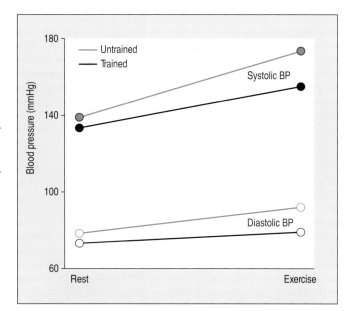

Figure 24.5 Modest reductions in blood pressure, both at rest and during exercise, have been reported with short courses of fitness training (Adapted from Clausen et al, Circulation 1969;**40**:143)

treatment. Fortunately, there have been a handful of studies that have looked at harder endpoints. All angiographic studies have shown either regression of atheroma, or a rate of progression that compares very favourably with the control groups (*Figure 24.6*). In terms of clinical events, however, the results have not been as impressive as, for example, those seen in cholesterol lowering studies. This difference is probably accounted for by a small number of deaths in the exercise groups, but this is offset by a greater improvement in symptoms such as angina in the exercise groups which, on balance, renders exercise therapy a valuable treatment in cardiac rehabilitation.

Chronic fatigue

This topic deserves mention in the context of exercise therapy in view of limited evidence for benefit in this condition. In a small study of mild exercise versus flexibility therapy, over 50% of subjects with chronic fatigue reported feeling better, or very much better in the exercise group. Improvement in the passive flexibility therapy group was very much less, leading to the conclusion that exercise may have a role to play in the treatment of chronic fatigue. It is not known whether improvement in subjects with this condition is continued in the long-term. Furthermore, many individuals whose symptom complex includes myalgia may not be able to undertake exercise programmes. Further research will be needed to answer these questions.

Summary

While clearly of benefit, it is important for the medical practitioner to be aware of the limits of exercise as a therapy. If an obese individual is prescribed exercise therapy, it would be very damaging if at a three month review, disappointment were expressed at a 1kg weight reduction since this is roughly what should be expected and should deserve encouragement. Similarly, there is probably little point in expecting exercise to reduce a total cholesterol of 7 mmol, or a blood pressure of 170/100 mmHg to the normal range, but rather the general benefits of exercise should be explained.

To date, it is not clear how much exercise or what type should be recommended. Although, conceptually, low grade, continuous aerobic exercise would seem sensible, a few studies have also shown that higher intensity exercise is equally beneficial. It would seem that it is the energy expended that is important and not the means of doing it. The optimal amount of exercise is not known, but a daily output of 300 kcal over and above daily living activity seems a reasonable recommendation. Casual advice to 'take exercise' is not helpful and, particularly in cardiac patients, exercise should be carefully prescribed. Well recognised methods using pulse rates, linked to perceived exertion and formal exercise testing are well described, and should be used. Such a goal is clearly not achievable if exercise is a chore, bolted on to the end of the day. Exercise should be incorporated into daily living and should ideally be enjoyable. The solution lies largely with the individual, but one cannot escape the conclusion that the process could be facilitated by local and national policies allowing better pedestrian and cycle facilities and any move toward public transport at the expense of the car should be applauded.

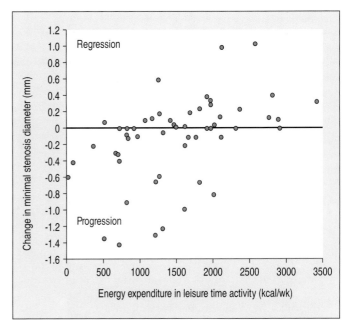

Figure 24.6 Progression of coronary lesions can be linked to the amount of leisure time physical activity performed (Reproduced from Hambrecht et al, Am J Coll Cardiol 1993;**22**:468)

Approximate energy expenditure for various activities

Activity		Energy output (kcal/min)
Sleeping and lying		1.0
Sitting		1.3
Standing		2.0
Walking	2 mph	2.8
	4 mph	5.0
Running	8 mph	15.0
Canoeing	4 mph	5.0
Horse riding	walk/gallop	6.5
Cycling	13 mph	7.5
Dancing		6.5
Gardening		7.5
Golf		5.0
Tennis		8.5
Football		9.0
Swimming	breast stroke	8.0
Squash		15.0
Skiing		15.0

The 15 grade scale for ratings of perceived exertion, the RPE scale (Borg GAV (1982)

Psychophysical bases of perceived exertion. *Med Sci Sports Exer* 14:377–81). Individuals indicate the degree of exertion involved in activity. Moderate activity is in the middle of the range. The expected heart rate approximates to the number on the scale multiplied by 10.

6	
7	very, very light
8	
9	very light
10	
11	fairly light
12	
13	somewhat hard
14	
15	hard
16	
17	very hard
18	
19	very, very hard
20	

Exercise prescription by heart rate
As a general rule, exercise should be prescribed at an intensity within the range 40–85% of functional capacity. For normal subjects, this is usually between 60 and 70% of functional capacity. In at risk groups, this is reduced to 40–60% in the first instance.

Heart rate reserve is calculated by subtracting the resting from the maximum heart rate. The product of the exercise intensity as a percentage and the heart rate reserve is added to the resting heart rate to obtain the training range of heart rate required, for example:

- maximum heart rate 160 bpm
- resting heart rate 70 bpm
- heart rate reserve 90 bpm
- 40% functional capacity = (0.4 x 90) + 70 = 106 bpm
- 80% functional capacity = (0.8 x 90) + 70 = 142 bpm

Further reading

Horgan JH (1996) Cardiac rehabilitation. *J Cardiovasc Risk* **3**: 139–140

O'Brien CP (1996) Exercise prescription; lessening the risk of physical activity. *J Cardiovasc Risk* **3**: 141–7

Zachwieja JJ (1996) Exercise as a treatment for obesity. *Endocrinol Metabol Clin N Am* **4**: 965–88

25 Nutrition, energy metabolism, and ergogenic supplements

Clyde Williams

Introduction

Athletes of the new millennium have access to a far greater range of foods than those who competed in the early Olympic Games and yet they share many of the same misunderstandings about the influence of food on performance. One of the shared myths is that there are "ergogenic supplements" that, when found, will allow athletes to train hard, recover quickly, and compete more successfully than their rivals. The reality is that if they exist, then they are probably pharmacological rather than nutritional supplements. Furthermore, in searching for such "quick fix foods" the contributions of commonly available foods to health and exercise performance are easily overlooked. The first and foremost nutritional need of athletes is for a well balanced diet, made up of a wide range of foods in sufficient quantity to cover their energy expenditure. Thereafter, they can adopt nutritional strategies to ensure that they can train, compete, and recover more successfully than they would if left to follow their own appetites and perceptions about what and when to eat.

Nutrition

A well balanced diet is one that derives at least 50% of its energy from carbohydrate containing foods (CHO), less than 35% from fats, and 12 to 15% from protein. However, within the population at large only endurance athletes and vegetarians have diets that match these recommendations (*Figures 25.1* and *25.2*). One of the myths that many modern athletes share with the Olympians of Antiquity is that increased meat (protein) intake helps develop strength. It is mainly the strength and power athletes who cling to this idea about the link between protein intake and increased strength. The reality is that athletes undertaking heavy daily training need only slightly more protein than that recommended for the general population. The daily protein requirements of most people are covered by an intake of about 1 g/kg body weight, whereas a protein intake of between 1.5 and 1.7 g/kg is sufficient for athletes undergoing heavy training. These amounts are less than the daily protein intakes of power athletes, which are often as high as 3 g/kg body mass.

The amount of food consumed should be sufficient to cover daily energy expenditure, but not be such that it results in a significant increase in body weight. A stable body weight is one indicator that an athlete is in energy balance, i.e. that energy intake is equal to energy expenditure. However,

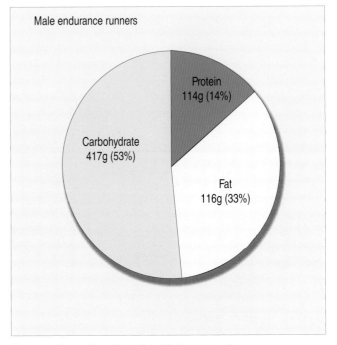

Figure 25.1 Composition of the daily food intake of male distance runners

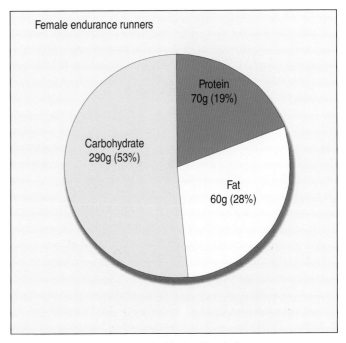

Figure 25.2: Composition of the daily food intake of female distance runners

energy balance should be assessed over several days rather than on a daily basis because of the fluctuations in energy intake and expenditure. When energy intake exceeds energy expenditure as a consequence of eating even a well balanced diet, the additional energy is stored and experienced as a gain in body weight.

"How much should I eat?" is as common a question among sportspeople as it is with the less active. The answer depends on their basal metabolic rate and their daily levels of physical activity. Basal metabolic rate (BMR) is the minimum amount of energy required to support life and it accounts for about 60% of our daily energy expenditure. It varies with age and can be estimated from body weight. One way of describing the energy cost of physical activity (PAL) is as multiples of BMR.

$$Physical\ Activity\ Level\ (PAL) = \frac{Total\ energy\ expended\ during\ 24\ hours}{Basic\ Metabolic\ Rate\ (BMR)\ over\ 24\ hours}$$

For example, people who are engaged in sedentary occupations have energy expenditures that are about 1.55 times their BMR; whereas, in sports involving prolonged heavy exercise, larger energy expenditures are necessary. At the top end of the range of daily energy expenditures are professional cyclists who achieve values of 3.3 times their basal metabolic rate when racing. Therefore, to maintain energy balance these athletes must eat large quantities of energy dense foods. For example, in the Tour De France, the professional cyclists have daily energy intakes of about 6500 kcal (27.17 MJ), increasing to about 9000 kcal (37.6 MJ) during the mountain section of the race. Their average daily energy intake is about double that of active healthy people (2500 kcal to 3000 kcal).

Energy metabolism

The main fuels for energy production are carbohydrates and fat. Protein plays only a very minor part as a fuel during exercise in well fed individuals. Carbohydrate is stored in the form of a glucose polymer (glycogen) in muscle and in liver. Liver glycogen provides glucose for brain metabolism and it also supplements glycogen metabolism in skeletal muscles during exercise (*Figure 25.3*). The average glycogen concentration in each kg of skeletal muscles is approximately 13 g and, in an adult man, muscle contributes about 40% to overall body mass. Therefore, the glycogen content of skeletal muscle is about 360 g and the energy yield from carbohydrate is approximately 4 kcal/g (16.7 kjoules/g). Thus, the energy equivalent of skeletal muscle glycogen is about 1440 kcal (6019 kjoules). In addition, the adult liver, weighing about 1.8kg, contains approximately 90 to 100 g of glycogen and so, in total, the energy equivalent of stored carbohydrate is equivalent to about 2000 kcal (8360 kjoules). There is approximately 3 g of water stored with every gram of glycogen, so any gain in body weight following a high carbohydrate diet is not entirely due to the increased storage of carbohydrate.

Fat is stored in adipose tissue cells in the form of triacylglycerides (triglycerides) and is far more plentiful than the body's carbohydrate stores. Lean men have about 15% of their body weight as fat, whereas the value for lean women is about 20%. Complete oxidation of fat yields the equivalent of 9 kcal/g (37.6 kjoules/g) and so the average 70 kg man (15% body fat) has approximately 94 500 kcal (~400 000 kjoules) of energy stored as fat. Thus the energy stored as carbohydrate is only 2% of the available energy stored as fat.

The metabolic degradation of fat and carbohydrate produces adenosine triphosphate (ATP), described as the 'energy currency

Formulae for calculating basal metabolic rate (BMR) for men and women

Age (years)	BMR of males obtained from:	BMR of females obtained from:
10 to 17	17.5 x W + 651	12.2 x W + 746
18 to 29	15.3 x W + 679	14.7 x W + 496
30 to 59	11.6 x W + 879	8.7 x W + 829

W = body weight in kg. BMR values obtained are in kcal/day
(From the 1985 FAO/WHO/UNO report)

Physical activity levels for different amounts of daily activity

	Type of daily physical activity level (PAL)		
	Light	**Moderate**	**Heavy**
Men	1.55 x BMR	1.78 x BMR	2.10 x BMR
Women	1.56 x BMR	1.64 x BMR	1.82 x BMR

(From the 1985 FAO/WHO/UNO report)

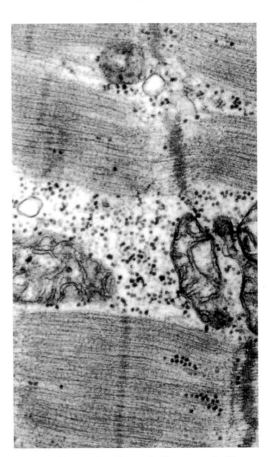

Figure 25.3 Electron photomicrograph of human muscle. The sample, obtained by percutaneous needle biopsy was taken before exercise to fatigue. The black dots are the glycogen granules dispersed between the myofibrils and mitochondria. Clear droplets of triglycerides are also visible although not as abundant as the glycogen granules

of life'. Almost every energy demanding physiological process uses ATP and, because it is not stored in large quantities, it has to be rapidly resynthesised. At rest, ATP resynthesis is achieved mainly by the oxidation of fat, with only a minor contribution from carbohydrate metabolism. Oxidation of fat and carbohydrate takes place in the mitochondria, which are like small cells within cells. The capacity for aerobic metabolism is directly related to the number of mitochondria in each muscle fibre. Muscle is made up of two populations of fibres. One is the slow contracting, slow fatiguing fibres (Type 1) that are generally rich in mitochondria, whereas the fast contracting, fast fatiguing fibres (Type 2) have relatively few mitochondria. The Type 1 fibres mainly resynthesise ATP by aerobic metabolism of fat and carbohydrate. In contrast, the Type 2 fibres (sprint fibres) rely almost entirely on the anaerobic degradation of glycogen to complement phosphocreatine (see below) in resynthesising ATP during exercise.

As we move from rest to exercise, ATP is used more rapidly to cover the energy demands of working skeletal muscles. During the onset of exercise, the rate of ATP production from the oxidation of fat and carbohydrate is too slow to match the rate at which ATP is used. This is largely a result of initial adjustments of the cardiovascular system to increased demands for oxygen delivery. Therefore, the oxidative contribution of the fat and carbohydrate to ATP production is temporarily inadequate. Fortunately, there are mechanisms in place to cover this temporary energy deficit, otherwise we would not have the ability to sprint nor change running speed as and when the occasion demands. We cope because muscle has a high energy compound called phosphocreatine (PCr) which has three times more potential energy than ATP. In energy-demanding cellular processes, ATP is reduced to ADP (adenosine diphosphate). The PCr rapidly converts ADP to ATP to allow the contractile activity in skeletal muscle to continue, during which time the contributions to ATP resynthesis from fat and carbohydrate gradually increase.

Carbohydrate metabolism helps cover some of the energy deficit at the start of exercise because the early steps in the degradation of muscle glycogen do not require oxygen. This is described as the anaerobic degradation of glycogen which provides three ATP rather than the 38 ATP following complete degradation. However, this smaller number of ATP are produced rapidly and so help PCr to quickly replace the ATP used by working skeletal muscles. The anaerobic or non-oxidative production of three ATP is accompanied by the formation of lactic acid (or more accurately, lactate and hydrogen ions). The appearance of lactate in the blood is often wrongly interpreted as energy production in the absence of cellular oxygen, rather than as reflecting the differential rates of aerobic and anaerobic production of ATP.

After several minutes of submaximal exercise, oxygen demand is met by oxygen delivery and ATP is produced by the oxidation of fat and carbohydrate. However, the relative contributions are dependent on a number of physiological conditions. The first is the exercise intensity relative to the individual's maximum capacity for oxygen consumption (VO$_2$max). At low relative exercise intensities (< 50%VO$_2$max), fat is the main fuel with only a minor contribution from carbohydrate metabolism. As exercise intensity increases, there is a greater contribution from carbohydrate metabolism and fatigue occurs when the stores of muscle glycogen are used up (*Figure 25.4*). However, the carbohydrate used during exercise is not confined to muscle glycogen because blood glucose derived from the liver also contributes to muscle metabolism, but mainly during the later stages of prolonged exercise.

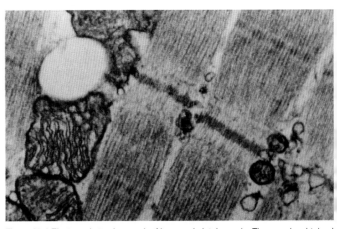

Figure 25.4 Electron photomicrograph of human skeletal muscle. The sample, obtained by percutaneous needle biopsy, was taken when the subject fatigued after two hours of cycling. The absence of glycogen granules provides supportive evidence for the strong association between glycogen depletion and fatigue

Long chain fatty acids are mobilised from adipose tissue cells and transported in loose combination with plasma albumin to working muscle, where they are taken up and either oxidised in mitochondria or stored as intramuscular triglycerides. Oxidation of long chain fatty acids produce about 140 ATP, whereas the oxidation of glycogen produces only 38 ATP. Intramuscular triglycerides contribute to muscle metabolism, especially when the delivery of plasma fatty acids is less than the capacity of muscle to oxidise them. Fat and carbohydrate act in concert with PCr to cover the ATP needs of skeletal muscle. The relative contributions of these two fuels are also influenced by the training status of the individual and the composition of the last meal. Endurance training increases the number of capillaries around each of the Type 1 fibres and their mitochondrial density. The consequence of this adaptation is that, during submaximal exercise, the endurance trained individuals will use more fat to cover their energy expenditure than the less well trained. As a result, the rate of glycogen degradation will be slower and so endurance capacity will increase.

A high carbohydrate meal consumed about three hours before exercise will also improve endurance capacity when compared with exercise time after fasting. The nature of the carbohydrate will influence the amount of fat metabolism before and during exercise. A meal containing high glycaemic index carbohydrates will raise plasma glucose and insulin concentrations and, as a consequence of the elevated insulin concentrations, fatty acid mobilisation from adipose tissue cells is inhibited. The decreased availability of fatty acids will be covered by an increase in carbohydrate metabolism in skeletal muscles with some contribution from intramuscular triglycerides. However, despite a reduction in fat metabolism during the early part of prolonged exercise, it appears not to compromise endurance capacity. Eating low glycaemic index carbohydrate pre-exercise meals does not depress fatty acid mobilisation, or utilisation during exercise. Paradoxically, there appears to be no obvious improvement in endurance capacity as a consequence of greater fat metabolism.

During brief high intensity exercise, such as sprinting, the limiting factor is not glycogen depletion, but probably the widespread cellular effects of a decrease in muscle pH. The capacity to perform repeated maximum sprints depends not only on delaying a severe reduction in muscle pH, but also on the muscle's ability to rapidly resynthesise PCr between sprints. When the intensity of each sprint is slightly less than maximum, after many more sprints depletion of muscle glycogen again becomes the limitation to further exercise. In a multiple-sprint sport, such as soccer, those players with low muscle glycogen concentrations run less than players with more adequate glycogen stores.

Nutritional strategies

Before exercise
Recognising the central role carbohydrate plays in energy metabolism during exercise, it is not surprising that nutritional strategies have been developed to increase muscle glycogen stores before exercise. The most effective and acceptable method of carbohydrate-loading is to decrease training three to four days before competition and increase the consumption of carbohydrate containing foods in each meal. A daily intake of about 9 to 10 g/kg body weight of carbohydrate is sufficient to increase muscle and liver glycogen stores prior to competition. Furthermore, a high carbohydrate meal eaten three to four hours before competition also helps to top up glycogen stores.

During exercise
Dehydration can cause fatigue during prolonged exercise just as effectively as depletion of muscle glycogen. Drinking well formulated carbohydrate-electrolyte solutions (i.e. several sports drinks) throughout exercise helps prevent severe dehydration and contributes to carbohydrate metabolism in working muscles, delaying the onset of fatigue (see *Chapter 23*). Sports drinks that provide carbohydrate at a rate of between 30 and 50 g/hour are effective in increasing endurance performance.

After exercise
Speed of recovery from exercise depends on how quickly muscle glycogen can be replaced and fluid balance restored. Muscle glycogen resynthesis is most rapid immediately after exercise, so drinking a carbohydrate-electrolyte solution (or eating high glycaemic index carbohydrate foods) after exercise will produce the maximum rate of glycogen resynthesis. The optimum amount of carbohydrate is 1 g/kg body weight, which is achieved by drinking about a litre of a sports drink containing 6 to 7% carbohydrate. However, consuming 50 g of carbohydrate every hour until the next meal appears to be a more practical recommendation. The overall carbohydrate intake during the recovery over a 24-hour period should be equivalent to about 10 g/kg body weight. Delaying the consumption of carbohydrate for two to three hours after exercise reduces the rate of glycogen resynthesis and delays the return of endurance fitness. When attempting to recover within 24 hours, food intake must be prescribed because an *ad libitum* intake will not provide sufficient carbohydrate to replace muscle glycogen, or restore energy balance.

Nutritional (ergogenic) supplements

Unfortunately, too many sportspeople are vulnerable to the advertising claims that supplements enhance performance. The most popular nutritional supplements are those shown , but there are many others that make claims without any supporting evidence, so these have not been included in this brief overview.

Vitamins and minerals
Vitamin and mineral supplementation is a common practice among many sportspeople, despite there being no good evidence to show that performance is enhanced following a period of supplementation of a well balanced diet with additional vitamins

---

Two menus for high carbohydrate diets

Breakfast

Weetabix (4)	Baked beans on thick sliced
Semi-skimmed milk	toast (3)
Crumpets (2) with honey	Low-fat spread (thinly spread)
Orange juice	Orange juice
Tea/coffee (preferably	Tea/coffee (preferably
decaffeinated)	decaffeinated

Mid-morning snack

Malt loaf	Digestive biscuits (2)
Low-fat spread (thinly spread)	Banana
Diet squash (1 pint)	Low-fat milkshake

Lunch

French bread	Wholemeal hoagie
Lean ham	Lean beef
Reduced-fat Cheddar	Low-fat spread (thinly spread)
Low-fat spread (thinly spread)	Tomato, lettuce, cucumber
Pickles	Packet of 'French Fries' crisps
Low-fat rice pudding (for	Low-fat fruit yoghurt
example, Müllerice®)	Diet squash/water
Pear	
Diet squash/water	

Mid-afternoon snack

Apple and banana	Currant bun
Diet squash/water	Tea/coffee (preferably
	decaffeinated)

Dinner

Roast chicken	Pasta with lean ham,
Mushrooms, onions, peas, and	mushrooms, onion, and cheese
mixed vegetables (stir-fried in a	sauce (made with
sweet and sour sauce)	semi-skimmed milk and a
Boiled basmati rice	cheese sauce packet mix)
Swiss roll and vanilla dairy	Bread roll
ice-cream	Bread and butter pudding
Tea/coffee (preferably	Tea/coffee (preferably
decaffeinated)	decaffeinated)

Supper

Fruit'n Fibre	Gingernut biscuits (5)
Semi-skimmed milk	Low-fat hot chocolate
Diet squash/water	

Energy 2944 kcal of which:	Energy 2804 kcal, of which:
Protein (183 g) 19%	Protein (112 g) 16%
Fat 15%	Fat 22%
Carbohydrate 65%	Carbohydrate 62%

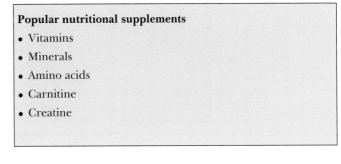

Popular nutritional supplements

- Vitamins
- Minerals
- Amino acids
- Carnitine
- Creatine

and minerals. However, the assumption that all athletes consume a diet containing a wide range of foods that provides sufficient energy to cover their energy expenditure is not always true. People who participate in sports with strict weight categories generally attempt to compete in a weight class that is lower than their normal training weight. Low energy intakes and high energy expenditures carry the potential threat of nutrient deficiency. This is particularly true for females who must pay particular attention to their intake of iron, calcium, and folic acid.

Amino acids

In addition to extra protein-containing foods, many strength athletes also supplement their diets with amino acids, especially those such as arginine, that stimulate an increased release of growth hormone. However, the growth hormone releasing effect of these amino acids is far less than that produced by exercise alone and too many strength athletes, and their coaches, mistakenly continue to extol the performance benefits of amino acid supplementation.

Branched-chain amino acids have also been suggested as a way of delaying "central fatigue". The central fatigue concept proposes that the rise in plasma-free tryptophan during prolonged exercise increases serotonin, one of the brain's neurotransmitters, which in turn decreases the drive to continue exercising. Branched-chain amino acids (valine, leucine, and isoleucine) share the same carrier mechanism for crossing the blood-brain barrier with tryptophan. Thus, the hypothesis is that raising the plasma concentration of branched-chain amino acids will result in competitive inhibition of tryptophan's transport across the blood-brain barrier and avoid large increases in serotonin. Ingesting branched-chain amino acids during prolonged exercise increases their plasma concentration and reduces the ratio of free tryptophan to branched-chain amino acids (*Figure 25.6*). Although the rate of perceived exertion is reduced, endurance performance is not improved with this amino acid supplementation.

Carnitine

Carnitine plays an essential role in fat metabolism. It is responsible for transporting fatty acids into mitochondria in skeletal muscles, where they undergo aerobic metabolism. The rationale for supplementing the diet with carnitine is that more fatty acids can be transported into mitochondria and this will result in increased fat metabolism. In turn, this reduces the rate at which the limited glycogen stores are used for energy metabolism and so delays the onset of fatigue. Muscle has more than enough endogenous carnitine, however, so it is not surprising that carnitine supplementation has not been shown to improve human endurance capacity.

Medium chain triacylglycerol

Medium chain triacylglycerols are more rapidly absorbed and oxidised than the long chain triacylglycerols that are obtained from dietary fat. Neither do they reduce gastric emptying and are rapidly oxidised, especially when ingested with carbohydrates. However, there is no clear evidence that low doses (~30 g) of this particular fat supplement improves performance. Higher doses cause gastrointestinal disturbances and, in some people, nausea and diarrhoea.

Creatine

In multiple-sprint sports, the rate of ATP resynthesis is more important than the capacity for energy production. The rapid resynthesis of ATP occurs as a result of the contributions from the degradation of PCr and glycogenolysis. Performance during a

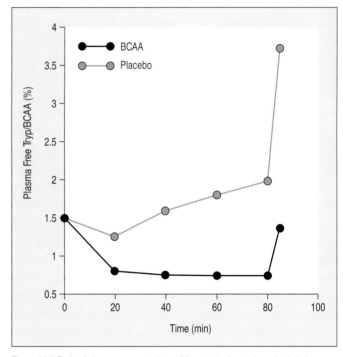

Figure 25.6 Ratio of plasma concentrations of free tryptophan to branched-chain amino acid (BCAA) during prolonged exercise following the ingestion of BCAA and placebo (From Blomstrand E, Hassmen P, Ek S, Ekblom B, Newsholme E (1997) Influence of ingesting a solution of branched-chain amino acids on the perceived exertion during exercise. Acta Physiol Scand **159**: 41–9)

series of maximum sprints, separated by recovery periods of no more than 30 seconds, decreases because there is not enough time for resynthesis of PCr. Creatine supplementation before exercise delays this decrease in performance by increasing the resynthesis of PCr. The main source of creatine is from foods containing meat or fish. However, creatine monohydrate is the supplement used and one gram is equivalent to the creatine content in 1 kg of fresh meat. In laboratory studies, the effective dose of creatine is 20 to 30 g/day for five to six days. Creatine supplementation at this level increases the pre-exercise PCr concentration, but about half is lost in urine. Lower doses of creatine also appear to influence performance during repeated sprints when recovery between sprints is longer than 60 seconds (*Figure 25.7*).

Caffeine and bicarbonate supplementation have also been shown to have performance enhancing effects under specific exercise conditions. However, neither of these are nutrients and do not cover any dietary deficiencies. In the doses shown to be effective, caffeine and bicarbonate supplementation act as pharmacological agents and do not have a legitimate role in the preparation for participation in, and recovery from, sport and exercise.

Metabolic ergogenic aids

- Caffeine
  - (but effective amounts are banned by the International Olympic Committee
- Bicarbonate
  - (but effective amounts cause unpleasant reactions

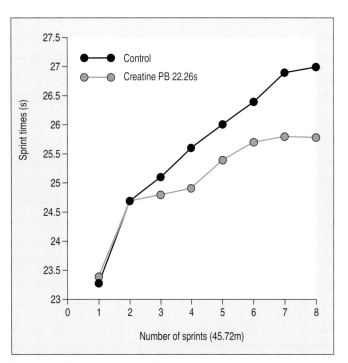

Figure 25.7 Influence of creatine supplementation (9 g/day for 5 days) on performance during sprint swimming (8 x 45.72 m (50 yards)) at intervals of 90 seconds (From Peyrebrune M, Nevill M, Donaldson F, Cosford D (1998) The effects of oral creatine supplementation on performance in single and repeated sprint swimming. J Sports Sci **16**: 271–9)

Summary

Apart from appropriate training, a high carbohydrate diet and an adequate fluid intake are the essential elements in the formula for successful preparation for the participation in, and recovery from, sport and exercise. Strategic supplementation of some nutrients, such as creatine, may be of benefit for participants in multiple-sprint sports.

26 The female athlete triad

Jane Gibson

Introduction

For many years, it has been recognised that some female athletes develop infrequent or absent menstruation (oligomenorrhoea and amenorrhoea respectively) while in training. Over the last ten to fifteen years, it has also been established that such athletes have low bone mineral density at certain important skeletal sites. More recently, it has been recognised that many of these women have inadequate nutritional intake or exhibit abnormal eating behaviour. These three features are now believed to be linked and comprise the "female athlete triad".

Incidence of menstrual abnormalities in athletes

Short luteal phases, anovulatory cycles, oligomenorrhoea, and amenorrhoea have all been described in athletes. Whereas secondary amenorrhoea occurs in only 5% of the general population, it is common in sports in which thinness may be an added advantage to performance. In these sports, there is increased pressure on young women to lose weight or to maintain an unrealistically low weight. Sometimes this may be because they will achieve faster times, for example, distance running, but in others it may be because of aesthetic appeal, for instance in gymnastics where the pre-pubertal female form has become accepted as normal. In some of the national squads of these sports, the incidence of menstrual abnormality approaches 100%. The term "athletic amenorrhoea" has now come into use to describe secondary amenorrhoea in athletes.

Causes of menstrual disturbance

There is no doubt that the aetiology of athletic amenorrhoea is multifactorial and some of the suggested causes are shown. However, there is emerging evidence that nutritional factors are a key element.

The role of eating disorders

Several reports have suggested that the calorie intake of amenorrhoeic athletes may be lower than that of eumenorrhoeic subjects and that restriction of energy intake may be linked causally to menstrual dysfunction. Several studies have reported lower mean daily energy intakes in amenorrhoeic runners compared to eumenorrhoeic runners. This difference may be up to 520 kcal/day and intakes as low as 1200 kcal/day are common.

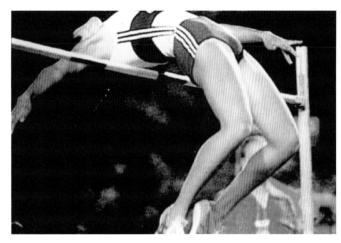

Figure 26.1

Categorisation of sports according to whether low body mass is likely to improve performance or increase marks obtained during performance

Low weight not of specific benefit to performance	Low weight likely to improve performance	Performance judged on aesthetic appeal	Competing in weight categories
Heavy weight rowing	Running middle	Gymnastics	Judo
Ball games, for example:	long	Gymnastics rhythmic	Martial arts
lacrosse	ultra	Figure skating	Rowing lightweight
hockey	cross-country	Ice dance	Weight-lifting
basketball	Orienteering	Dancing competitive	Wrestling
netball	Race-walking	ballet	
tennis	Jumping	Body-building	
Golf	Pole vault	Swimming synchro	
Sprinting	Rowing cox	Diving	
Field events (throwing)	Jockeys flat racing		
Contact sports	Cycling		
Swimming	Triathlon		
Water polo	Climbing competitive		
Skiing	Windsurfing Olympic		
Speed skating	Sailing some classes		
Luge/bobsleigh			

Anorexia nervosa and bulimia are both associated with amenorrhoea, or other alterations in menstrual function, and it seems likely that the same occurs in athletes. Surveys of gymnasts, endurance runners, ballet dancers and ice skaters have all shown consistently high rates of abnormal eating behaviours, such as severe dieting, purging, vomiting, and fasting. A 1989 survey of female ice skaters found that 48% had eating questionnaire scores in the range of clinical anorexia nervosa. In dancers, self-reported anorexia or bulimia ranges from 11% in highly select dancers to 33% in regional, national, or university dance companies. Although more common in such sports, abnormal eating behaviours can be found in athletes from any discipline.

Eating disorders are associated with considerable morbidity, and even mortality, and are associated with reduced levels of performance. However, it is the long-term effects on bone mineralisation due to amenorrhoea that are particularly concerning.

The effects of menstrual irregularity on bone

In general, athletes have a greater bone density than their sedentary counterparts, due to a combination of ground reaction forces during weight-bearing and mechanical strain produced by muscular pull. Not all female athletes have high bone density. The surprising finding has been the extent to which mineral bone density (BMD) is different in amenorrhoeic athletes compared to either sedentary controls or eumenorrhoeic peers.

Menstruation and bone density of non weight-bearing bones
Studies on amenorrhoeic runners compared with either eumenorrhoeic runners or sedentary controls have been consistent in showing lumbar BMD to be 10–20% lower in those with amenorrhoea. A linear relationship exists between vertebral BMD and menstrual history such that those who are amenorrhoeic have, on average, a mean BMD 17% lower than those who have always had regular periods. Athletes with less severe menstrual disruption have intermediate bone densities (*Figure 26.2*).

The effect of hypo-oestrogenism on the lumbar spine may not be as marked in athletes whose sports require considerable back strength (for example, rowers, gymnasts) possibly due to the beneficial effects of high muscular strain imposed on the spine.

Menstruation and bone density of weight-bearing bones
It was expected that the remodelling effects of weight-bearing exercise would offset any detrimental effects of amenorrhoea, but recent studies have shown a difference of 15–20% in BMD in various femoral regions in amenorrhoeic runners compared to their eumenorrhoeic peers. Not only is the difference in BMD similar to that found in the spine, but there also seems to be a linear relationship between severity of menstrual irregularity and BMD of the femur. However, the BMD of the femur in these athletes is closer to that of sedentary controls than in the spine, suggesting that, to some extent, regular running can offset bone loss due to amenorrhoea (*Figure 26.3*).

Mechanism of reduced bone density in amenorrhoeic athletes

Normal bone metabolism requires an intact hypothalamic-pituitary-ovarian axis. Oestrogen prevents bone resorption and

Non-pathological factors that may contribute to the development of menstrual dysfunction in athletes

- Low body mass
- Low body fat
- Restricted nutritional intake
- Eating disorders
- Younger age
- Late menarche
- Previous menstrual irregularity
- High training volume or intensity
- Psychological and social stresses
- Vegetarianism
- Non-parous

Those women with the greatest number of risk factors are the most likely to develop menstrual dysfunction

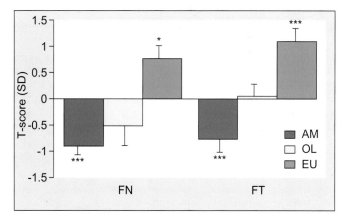

Figure 26.2 Bone mineral density of the proximal femur of 50 endurance-trained female runners compared to the young peak bone mass according to a standard reference range (Hologic Inc). This is known as the T-score and is expressed in standard deviations above or below the mean.

This shows the approximate linear relationship between number of menstrual cycles per year and bone density.

AM amenorrhoeic (0–3 cycles per year)
OL oligomenorrhoeic (4–10 cycles per year)
EU eumenorrhoiec (11–13 cycles per year)

FN neck of femur
FT trochanteric region of proximal femur

t-test compares each group with the Hologic range
*p<0.02, **o<0.01, ***p<0.001

decreases remodelling, whereas progesterone promotes bone formation and accelerates remodelling. Normally, bone resorption and formation are "coupled" so that appropriate remodelling can occur as required. In the presence of low levels of oestrogen and progesterone, resorption increases and since bone formation is insufficient to compensate, there is a net loss of bone mineral. Anovulation or a short luteal phase have been associated with bone mineral losses of up to 4% per annum.

It has been suggested that the principal defect is a reduction in bone formation rather than an increased resorption. High serum cortisol levels and low Insulin-like Growth Factor-1 (IGF-1) levels are known to be associated with reduced bone formation and these states have been found both in endurance athletes and anorexia nervosa. In particular, biochemical abnormalities are associated with an energy deficient state, such as occurs in amenorrhoeic athletes and anorexic patients (see below) and this has focussed even more attention on the role of eating habits.

Consequences of the female athlete triad

The worry is that failure to achieve maximum potential bone density at important skeletal sites will increase the risk of early osteoporosis and fracture. As yet there is no direct evidence for this, but, even in the short-term, such athletes do appear to have a higher incidence of musculoskeletal injury, particularly stress fractures. An osteoporotic fracture of the neck of humerus has been reported in a thirty-year-old runner with proven low bone density, and osteoporotic fracture is common in patients with anorexia nervosa. Lifetime risk of osteoporosis is related to peak bone mass and unless there is "catch-up" of bone mineralisation in these athletes later in life, they are likely to have a higher risk of osteoporosis than the rest of the population.

Can loss in bone density catch up?

Short-term studies over 12–24 months have shown improvements in lumbar spine BMD of 2–5% per year in athletes who regain menses either due to a reduction in training or a gain in weight. In one medium-term study over eight years, bone density of the lumbar spine in previously amenorrhoeic athletes remained at 84% of the eumeorrhoeic athlete value despite return of menstruation. Those with previous intermittent oligoamenorrhoea remained at an intermediate position of 94.7% of the eumenorrhoeic value. Cross-sectional studies on premenopausal veteran runners aged 40 years and over have also shown that while BMD of the femur is relatively preserved in those with a history of amenorrhoea, lumbar spine BMD remains lower than expected.

Thus, although all the short-term studies suggest that small improvements in BMD may occur in some regions of the skeleton when menstruation returns, these gains may be short-lived. If sufficient trabeculae are lost, it may be impossible to recalcify fully these areas of bone. If this is happening, early intervention to prevent irreversible bone loss will be required, but more studies with higher numbers of subjects are needed to confirm these suspicions.

Treatment of the female athlete triad

Prevention is likely to yield greater benefits than treatment. However, this is particularly difficult in athletes. Reduction in training levels is unlikely to be a possibility, although some benefit

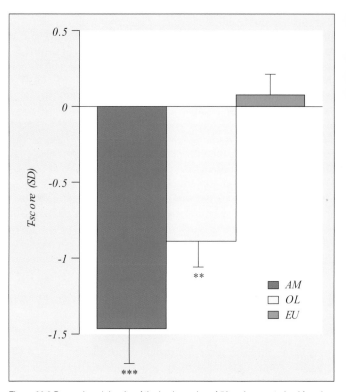

Figure 26.3 Bone mineral density of the lumbar spine of 50 endurance-trained female runners compared to the young peak bone mass according to a standard reference range (Hologic Inc). This is known as the T-score and is expressed in standard deviations above or below the mean.

This shows the approximate linear relationship between number of menstrual cycles per year and bone density.

AM amenorrhoeic (0–3 cycles per year)
OL oligomenorrhoeic (4–10 cycles per year)
EU eumenorrhoiec (11–13 cycles per year)

t-test compares each group with the Hologic range
*p<0.02, **p<0.01, ***p<0.001

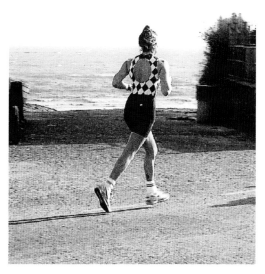

Figure 26.4

may be obtained by taking a fresh look at training content. Weight gain is usually strongly resisted and the use of pharmacological agents (particularly sex steroid hormones) is often viewed unfavourably because of worry about weight gain, emotional disturbance, or breast tenderness. Persuading athletes to admit to eating disorders is also difficult.

How should this triad be tackled? The first step is to increase awareness among all those who come into contact with female athletes. This includes national sports institutes, governing sports bodies, coaches, primary care physicians, sports doctors, orthopaedic surgeons, parents, and the athletes themselves. Proactive screening of athletes for menstrual irregularity and abnormal eating habits often helps to identify problems early and allows a management plan to be initiated.

Treatment should be aimed at improving nutritional parameters and normalising menstrual cycles. Additional psychological factors should also be addressed (*Figure 26.6*). If normal menstrual function does not return within 6 months despite optimisation of all other parameters, pharmacological intervention should be considered. There are various options available.

Oral contraceptive pill (OCP)

Athletes who have been on the OCP appear to have preserved BMD. However, its use to treat proven low BMD in amenorrhoeic athletes has not been firmly established. The OCP selected should contain full dose oestrogens. Progesterone-only pills and the "mini-pill" should be avoided.

Hormone replacement therapy (HRT)

A recent pilot study of oral HRT in athletes gave some support for its use, although side effects of weight gain and breast tenderness may present a problem. Its use requires regular monitoring of BMD and it should be withdrawn as soon as circumstances allow. Unopposed oestrogens must be avoided.

Specific oestrogen receptor modulators (SERMs)

These non-hormonal agents have recently come onto the market and are likely to become an alternative therapeutic option for the prevention and treatment of postmenopausal osteoporosis. They bind to oestrogen receptors on bone and have been shown to improve BMD. As they are not oestrogens, they appear to lack some of the risks normally associated with oestrogen therapy, such as breast cancer and deep vein thrombosis. They have not yet been fully evaluated.

Calcitonin

Calcitonin nasal spray has been used with some benefit, but it is not readily available at present and its use requires further evaluation.

Calcium and vitamin D supplementation

Supplementation with high doses of calcium and/or vitamin D has been disappointing. Although it does not prevent further reductions in BMD associated with ongoing amenorrhoea, it should not be ignored as an adjunct to therapy. Dietary calcium intake should also be optimised.

Musculoskeletal consequences of athletic amenorrhoea

- Increased frequency and duration of musculoskeletal injury
- Increased risk of stress fractures
- Low bone mineral density
- Fractures
- Possible risk of early osteoporosis

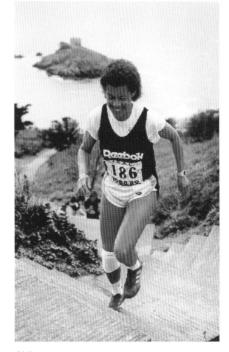

Figure 26.5

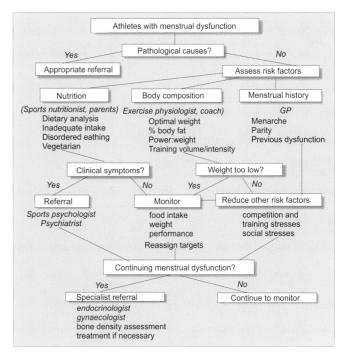

Figure 26.6 Flow diagram for assessment of athletes with menstrual dysfunction by clinicians. Management requires team approach and suggestions for personnel are given at relevant stages, if not already part of decision-making. No stages are mutually exclusive.

References

Drinkwater BL, Nilson K, Chesnut CH, Bremner WJ, Shainholtz S, Southworth MB (1984) Bone mineral content of amenorrhoeic and eumenorrhoeic athletes. *N Engl J Med* **311**: 277–81

Drinkwater BL, Nilson K, Ott S, Chesnut CH (1986) Bone mineral density after resumption of menses in amenorrhoeic athletes. *JAMA* **256**: 380–2

Drinkwater BL, Bremner B, Chesnut CH (1990) Menstrual history as a determinant of current bone density in young athletes. *JAMA* **263**: 545–8

Further reading

American College of Sports Medicine (1997) American College of Sports Medicine stand on the female athlete triad. *Med Sci Sports Exerc* **29**: i–ix

Gibson JH (1998) Exercise and the Skeleton. In: Harries M, Williams C, Stanish WD, Micheli LJ, eds. *Oxford Textbook of Sports Medicine*, 2nd edn. Oxford Medical Publications, Oxford

Wilson JH (1994) Nutrition, physical activity and bone health in women. *Nutr Res Rev* **7**: 67–91

Useful organisations

Womensport International, PO Box 227, Lawson, New South Wales 2783, Australia

---

Treatment options for athletic amenorrhoea

- Oral contraceptive pill
- Hormone replacement therapy
- Intranasal calcitonin
- Calcium supplementation
- ?Bisphosphonates
- ?Specific oestrogen receptor modulators (SERMs)

The most appropriate management strategy is to encourage resumption of the normal menstrual cycle by reduction of precipitating risk factors. Treatment should commence within six months of onset of amenorrhoea to avoid rapid loss of bone mineral

Index